The British Medical Association
FAMILY DOCTOR GUIDE *to*
DEPRESSION

The British Medical Association

FAMILY DOCTOR GUIDE *to*

DEPRESSION

Dr. Kwame McKenzie

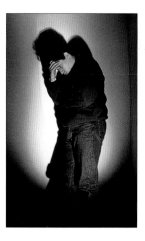

MEDICAL EDITOR
Dr. Tony Smith

A DORLING KINDERSLEY BOOK

IMPORTANT

This book is not designed as a substitute for personal medical advice but as a supplement to that advice for the patient who wishes to understand more about his/her condition.

Before taking any form of treatment **YOU SHOULD ALWAYS CONSULT YOUR MEDICAL PRACTITIONER.**

In particular (without limit) you should note that advances in medical science occur rapidly and some of the information contained in this book about drugs and treatment may very soon be out of date.

PLEASE NOTE

The author regrets that he cannot enter into any correspondence with readers.

DORLING KINDERSLEY

LONDON, NEW YORK, AUCKLAND, DELHI,
JOHANNESBURG, MUNICH, PARIS AND SYDNEY

[DK] www.dk.com

Senior Editors Nicki Lampon, Mary Lindsay
Senior Designers Jan English, Sarah Hall
Production Controller Elizabeth Cherry

Managing Editor Martyn Page
Managing Art Editor Bryn Walls

Produced for Dorling Kindersley Limited by
Design Revolution, Queens Park Villa,
30 West Drive, Brighton, East Sussex BN2 2GE
Editorial Director Ian Whitelaw
Art Director Becky Willis
Editor Julie Whitaker
Designer Andrew Easton

Published in Great Britain in 2000 by
Dorling Kindersley Limited,
9 Henrietta Street, London WC2E 8PS

2 4 6 8 10 9 7 5 3 1

A CIP catalogue record for this book is available from the British Library

ISBN 07513 08455

Reproduced by Colourscan, Singapore
Printed in Hong Kong by Wing King Tong

Contents

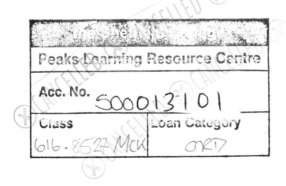

Introduction

We all have low moods from time to time. For instance, if a relationship breaks up we may feel shocked, we may cry, go off our food, get angry and irritable, sleep poorly and get tetchy and anxious.

Usually, the mood passes after a few days and we get back to our normal way of living. We may say that we have been 'depressed', 'down in the dumps', 'fed up' or have had the 'blues'.

But low moods like this are not what doctors call depression. Instead, they use the term to describe a more severe illness that a person has had for at least a few weeks, affecting the body as well as the mind.

It can come on for no reason at all and may sometimes be life threatening. No single symptom indicates whether you have just a low mood or what some people call 'clinical depression'. Many of the symptoms are similar; however, when you are depressed they are usually more intense and go on for longer.

A simple rule of thumb is that you should seek help if your low mood affects all parts of your life, lasts for two weeks or more or brings you to the

GETTING HELP
Family doctors are very experienced at dealing with depression. With their help, in the form of counselling, medication or other advice, most people will feel better.

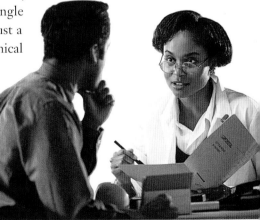

7

point of thinking about suicide. Try to remember that depression is an illness that can be treated successfully and you will feel better in time.

Ninety per cent of people with depression are treated by their GP and you shouldn't worry that he or she will think it a sign of weakness. Family doctors have years of experience in dealing with depression and are trained to diagnose and treat it. They may prescribe tablets but will probably also tell you about self-help organisations, counselling and psychotherapy or relaxation techniques. You may get advice on ways of decreasing your stress levels or coming to terms with a bereavement or other loss. GPs are a mine of information.

But, if you do not feel that you can talk to your doctor, talk with a friend. You will be surprised how many people have experience of depression, either first hand or because they know someone who has been depressed. They may be able to give you support and advice but, even if they just listen, talking to someone usually helps.

HOW COMMON IS DEPRESSION?

Many famous people have suffered from depression, including Abraham Lincoln, Queen Victoria and Winston Churchill, who called depression his 'black dog'. Many writers and actors have suffered from depression, and the comedian Spike Milligan has written a book – *Depression and How to Survive It* – about his depressive illness.

There has been an increase in the rates of depression over the last 40 years, which may be the result of the way we live our lives now. For many people the world is becoming increasingly stressful, and stress can lead to depression. Increases

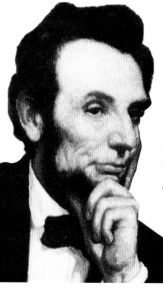

HEAD OF STATE
Abraham Lincoln is just one of the many well-known figures to have suffered a disorder that affects an ever-growing number of people.

in divorce rates, crime rates, longer working hours for some people and unemployment for others are just some of the factors that make life a strain for those affected.

Where we live may influence our risk of depression, too. One study showed that people who live in an inner-city area are twice as likely to be depressed as those who live in the Hebrides. Although it has proved difficult to find an exact reason for this, it is clear that your environment is an important factor in your risk of developing depression.

The good news is that no matter what the cause of depression it can be treated and treated effectively. Most people who are depressed and get treatment get better.

Facts about Depression

Anyone, of any age, can suffer from depression, although more women than men are affected.

- At least one in five adults will suffer from depression in their lifetime.
- Each year doctors diagnose two million cases in the UK.
- On average, each GP in the UK sees one patient with depression every day.
- Depression affects all age groups.
- Women are diagnosed as suffering from depression twice as often as men.

KEY POINTS

- Low moods are thought of as depression if they persist and affect all parts of your life.
- Depression is common.
- Depression can be treated effectively.

What is depression?

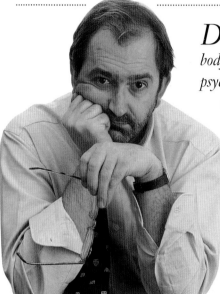

Depression is an illness of mind and body. Most people have both physical and psychological symptoms, but their exact nature will vary from one person to another. Different symptoms will be more or less prominent in each person's illness.

Some people report no symptoms of depression at all but begin behaving in an unusual way – for example, one previously law-abiding woman who came to my clinic had started shop-lifting when she became depressed.

PHYSICAL AND MENTAL
Depression can affect both the mind and the body, but individuals experience various combinations of symptoms.

PSYCHOLOGICAL SYMPTOMS

Despite the use of the label depression, not everyone with this illness feels low. Some are anxious, some say they are emotionally numb and some have no mood changes but come to their doctor with unexplained physical symptoms or with a change in behaviour. The more common psychological symptoms include the following.

LOW MOOD

In depression, low mood is much more intense than the way you feel when you are disappointed or just fed up. It is a persistent feeling of sadness, emptiness, loss and dread. Some say it is like living with a cloud over you,

Symptoms of Depression

The psychological symptoms of depression range from a sense of sadness or anxiety to severe delusions, whilst physical effects can include insomnia and weight loss.

PSYCHOLOGICAL SYMPTOMS

- Low mood
- Loss of interest in things you used to enjoy
- Anxiety
- Emotional numbness
- Depressive thinking
- Concentration and memory problems
- Delusions – see p.15
- Hallucinations
- Suicidal impulses

PHYSICAL SYMPTOMS

- Sleep problems – difficulty getting to sleep, waking up early or sleeping too much
- Mental and physical slowing
- Increase or decrease in appetite
- Increase or decrease in weight
- Loss of interest in sex
- Tiredness
- Constipation
- Menstrual period irregularities

and it takes over every part of your life. In moderate or severe depression, low mood is often worse in the morning and improves slightly during the day – though it never goes. This is called diurnal variation. Low mood makes it impossible to enjoy anything and you may even lose interest in your hobbies. Nothing brings you pleasure. Doctors call this symptom anhedonia.

In some milder cases, low mood may be worse in the evenings than in the mornings, and there may be the odd good day. However, these are outnumbered by the bad ones. If depression is mild you may be able to enjoy other people's company – though without stimulation you would soon become disenchanted again.

With the low mood comes a tendency to cry more often, with the slightest upset or even with no upset at all.

11

ANXIETY

When we feel threatened, a hormone called adrenaline is released and blood is directed to our muscles and brain so that we can think quickly and flee if we need to. We feel on edge, jumpy and tense but, if nothing happens, the feeling passes off in a few minutes. In someone who is depressed, these anxious feelings can last for months. Some people wake in the morning in a state of high anxiety because they dread the day ahead. Anxiety can outweigh low mood and be the most prominent symptom in depression. If you are in a state of anxiety you may find that you get irritable and snap a lot, which is obviously difficult for other people to live with as well as for you.

EMOTIONAL NUMBNESS

Some people who are severely depressed say they feel like they have completely lost their emotions, and this is one of the most distressing symptoms of depression. You feel numb. You cannot cry and feel like there are no tears left. You may not feel that you are part of the world because you do not think you have feelings. You may even feel distant and unfeeling about people very close to you, like your partner, family or children.

DEPRESSIVE THINKING

Your thinking changes when you are suffering from depression. You see the world differently and everything appears in a negative light. This distorted view simply reinforces the depression.

You may blame yourself for unfortunate events more than you should while not allowing yourself to take credit for things you have done well. The good things that you have done throughout your life are forgotten, while the bad things are vividly remembered and are blown up out of all proportion.

You may find yourself concentrating on the negative detail and ignoring the bigger picture. To take an extreme example, someone who had passed an exam with 99 per cent might ignore the good result and concentrate on the one per cent that they got wrong.

You may also start jumping to negative conclusions and jumping to general conclusions from single events. For instance, a model I once treated thought that she was ugly and everyone hated her because a man who passed her in the street gave her a funny look.

These sorts of negative thinking patterns undermine you. They lead to worry, a lack of confidence and feelings of worthlessness, and your world becomes full of gloomy thoughts, self-doubt and anxieties. As a result, you feel more depressed or anxious and so a vicious circle is set up.

VICIOUS CIRCLE
In her job as a secretary, Carrie's depression causes her to focus on the things that go wrong, and she becomes increasingly depressed.

Case History: **NEGATIVE THINKING**

Carrie is a secretary; her boss is late for the train and on his way out says, 'Could you type this report up for me, I have made a few corrections'.
Carrie is depressed, and because of this she thinks she is a failure. She believes that she has to correct the report because she is bad at her job.

Carrie then becomes more depressed because she has the unreasonable expectation that she must be perfect in her job if she is to enjoy her life.

In reality, she is good at her job, but she does not think so. She concentrates on the little things that go wrong rather than the big things that go right. She forgets the fact that she was given a pay rise because her company values her so much. She also ignores the fact that her boss is known to be indecisive and always changes reports that he has written. She concentrates on the negative details and jumps to a general conclusion based on a single incident – and this makes her more depressed.

While she is typing the report another thought comes to her: 'Could the boss be late because he had to correct my sloppy work? If the deal falls through it will be all my fault!' She blames herself for things that are not her fault, which fuels her depression.

The Elements of Depressive Thinking

Depressive thinking makes a person see the world in a negative light. There are three elements to depressive thinking:

- Negative thoughts, for example 'I am a failure at work'.
- High, unreasonable expectations, for example 'I cannot be happy unless everyone likes me and thinks I am good at my job'.
- Mistakes in thinking, for example:

  (a) Jumping to negative conclusions.

  (b) Focusing on negative details of a situation and ignoring the good bits.

  (c) Coming to a general conclusion on the basis of a single incident.

  (d) Coming to the conclusion that things that are nothing to do with you are your fault.

CONCENTRATION AND MEMORY PROBLEMS

If you are consumed by worries and depressive thoughts it can be difficult to think about anything else. You may find it difficult to concentrate and this leads to problems. You have to concentrate on something to remember it, so it is not surprising that poor concentration and memory problems go together.

Problems with concentration also lead to indecision and inattention; you may feel muddled and confused. These symptoms can be so severe as to be mistaken for dementia.

DELUSIONS AND HALLUCINATIONS

If you should become severely depressed, your thinking can become so distorted that you lose touch with reality. Your mind can start playing tricks on you and you may even fear that you are going mad. You are not; you are severely depressed and will get better with treatment. Delusions can occur in severe depression; thankfully (because they are so distressing) they are rare.

A delusion is a false belief that is held unshakeably by the person who has it. In depression, delusions reflect and reinforce the depressed mood, as happened with James whom I treated some time ago. He believed that he should give himself up to the police because he had mistakenly left a shop without paying for an apple five years previously. He thought that the police were looking for him and that there was no way out. He believed that he had brought shame on his family and was worthless. It was impossible to make him believe that he was not public enemy number one, that anyone could make a mistake and that no one would be bothered about it.

Other people believe they are the most wicked person in the world or that people want to get rid of them because they are so bad. Some people believe that they have no money at all; others that they are decaying or even that they are dead. There are as many different types of delusion as there are ideas in the human mind, but all of them reflect the depressed mood and depressive thinking.

Whereas delusions are false thoughts, hallucinations involve perceiving things that are not real – usually sounds. For example, some severely depressed people hear voices when there is no one there. The voices sound like people in the room talking to them and are frighteningly real. The voices may criticise them or tell them they are bad. The voices reinforce the depression. Some people see or smell things that are not there, but this is rarer.

SUICIDAL IMPULSES

When you are in the depths of depression the past looks bad and full of mistakes, the present is awful and you dread the future. Some people come to the conclusion that life is not worth living, that everyone would be better off without them and that they should take their own life.

Many depressed people think about suicide – even if it is just a passing thought. Many do not actually contemplate committing suicide but go to bed at night hoping that they will not wake up in the morning, and so get away from the terrible torture of living.

Most people decide they cannot do it, perhaps because it would be too drastic, because of the effect it would have on their family or because of religious beliefs. Some people come to the conclusion that they have not done it because they are cowards, and this makes them feel even more ashamed and depressed.

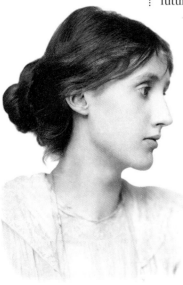

TORMENTED AUTHOR
Severe depression can lead to suicidal tendencies. The author Virginia Woolf suffered from severe depression and, at the age of 59, drowned herself.

If you think about suicide you are at risk of doing it. Get help urgently: see a GP, go to an accident and emergency department or call the Samaritans. Depression is treatable.

PHYSICAL SYMPTOMS

Depression can cause a number of physical symptoms. Those people affected often come to the conclusion that they have a physical illness because they feel so tired and off-colour or are in pain.

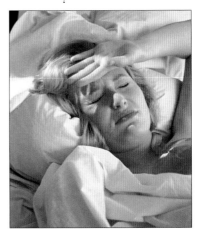

SLEEP PROBLEMS

Sleep problems are common in depression and are sometimes partially to blame for the tiredness that may be experienced. If you are suffering from moderate or severe depression you may wake up in the morning hours earlier than usual and then find it impossible to get back to sleep. All depressed people can find it difficult to get to sleep because they worry and may suffer from broken nights – waking up a number of times before the morning.

TROUBLED SLEEP
The worries and unpleasant thoughts that accompany depression can often cause a person to wake in the early hours of the morning.

MENTAL AND PHYSICAL SLOWING

If you are depressed you may feel like a machine that is seizing up. You feel tired all the time, it is hard to perform everyday chores, everything is an effort and it seems as if everything is slowed down. Your speech may be slow and monotonous and you may even move slowly. Doctors call this psychomotor retardation.

Sometimes body functions slow down or seize up as well. You may find that you have a dry mouth or that you become constipated; some women stop having periods or their periods may become irregular.

LOSS OF APPETITE

When you are depressed you can lose quite a lot of weight. Food seems unappetising and bland and you don't even feel hungry. Some people with severe depression completely stop eating and drinking, but this is rare.

REVERSE PHYSICAL SYMPTOMS

Instead of the normal physical symptoms of depression such as poor sleep, loss of appetite and loss of weight, some people have what are known as reverse physical symptoms. They sleep more, have a bigger appetite and gain weight. If you feel low in mood and have these symptoms you should see your doctor.

OTHER PHYSICAL SYMPTOMS

Depression can produce just about any physical symptom. Pain and a feeling of pressure are common, most often affecting the head, face, back, chest and gut.

People frequently come to hospital accident and emergency departments complaining of chest pain and worrying that something is wrong with their hearts, when in fact they are suffering from depression. The pain is real but is caused by depression, and there is nothing wrong with their hearts.

SEX

Many people go off sex when they are depressed. There are many reasons for this. Some people do not feel able to fulfil a physically loving relationship when they are emotionally numb. Other people feel so negative about themselves that they cannot relax. These psychological problems can lead to physical problems: men may find it difficult to get an erection and women may find that they are dry and that intercourse is painful. Many people who are depressed cannot say why but just do not feel interested in sex.

'SMILING' DEPRESSION

Not everyone with depression feels low – some people say they do not feel depressed but go to their GP with bodily symptoms such as pain, headache or tiredness that point to depression. Physical examination and investigation do not reveal a physical cause for their illness, and the only treatment that works is antidepressant medication. It may be that their subconscious mind is playing tricks on them and does not allow their conscious mind to admit that they feel depressed.

WHAT CAUSES THE SYMPTOMS?

The symptoms of depression may be caused by low levels of certain chemicals in the brain. To understand why this might be, we need to look at how the brain works. It is made up of billions of nerve cells. It can take hundreds of these cells to carry out an action, even to think about doing something. In order for the cells to work together they have to communicate with each other and they do this by releasing chemicals called neurotransmitters.

Between the end of one nerve cell and the next there is a small space called the synapse. The first nerve cell communicates with the next nerve cell by releasing neurotransmitters into the synapse. These neurotransmitters attach to the next nerve cells and so pass on the message.

Studies have shown that in people who are suffering from depression three important neurotransmitters – dopamine, serotonin and noradrenaline – are in short

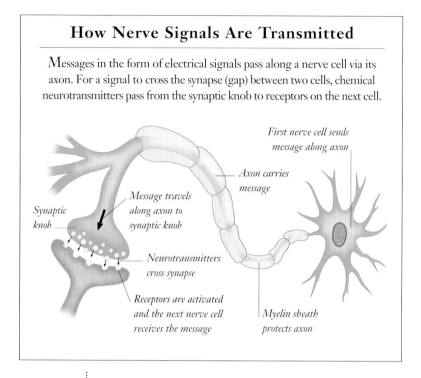

How Nerve Signals Are Transmitted

Messages in the form of electrical signals pass along a nerve cell via its axon. For a signal to cross the synapse (gap) between two cells, chemical neurotransmitters pass from the synaptic knob to receptors on the next cell.

First nerve cell sends message along axon

Axon carries message

Message travels along axon to synaptic knob

Synaptic knob

Neurotransmitters cross synapse

Receptors are activated and the next nerve cell receives the message

Myelin sheath protects axon

supply. The levels are low in synapses, and this leads to faulty brain communication and message passing that may be the cause of depressive symptoms.

Nobody knows what causes these low levels of chemicals. Scientists do not know whether they cause the depressed mood or are caused by the depressed mood. It may be that low levels of neurotransmitters are caused by stress and then they lead to depression. Antidepressant drugs work by increasing the levels of these chemicals.

THE ROLE OF HORMONES

Hormones may be important in causing the symptoms of depression. We have seen that adrenaline causes

20

anxiety, and the role of female hormones in depression is discussed on p.25. Another hormone that may be important in depression is cortisol.

Cortisol is important in our body's reaction to stress. Cortisol has wide-ranging actions on all parts of our body metabolism so that we are ready for action in an emergency. It changes our immune reaction, our kidney function and the levels of fats and sugars in our blood. Its release, which is controlled by the pituitary gland in the brain, does not follow the normal pattern in people who are depressed. In healthy people, cortisol is usually released in large quantities in the morning and in diminishing amounts throughout the day, whereas in some depressed people its release is the same all day long. Nobody knows whether this leads to depression or is the result of it, but cortisol does affect the levels of neurotransmitters in the brain.

Changing levels of cortisol in the body have led to a test for depression, but it is not that sensitive and only works in about three out of 10 people. The test works best in those who are suffering from serious depression with physical symptoms.

KEY POINTS

- Depression has physical as well as mental symptoms.
- Symptoms vary from person to person.
- Anyone who thinks about suicide is at risk of doing it and should seek help urgently.

Causes of depression

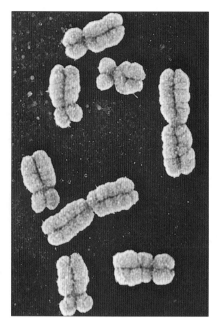

THE GENETIC FACTOR
Found in chromosomes in every cell in our bodies, the genes that we inherit from our parents can influence the likelihood that we will suffer from depression.

The questions most often asked by people who are depressed are 'Why me?' and 'Why now?'. Sometimes there is an obvious cause for depression, such as bereavement, but often there is not.

To complicate the question of the causes of depression still further, depression does not affect everyone who is bereaved, loses their job or becomes ill. We all have our strengths and weaknesses. Some people may be more at risk of depression than others but, given the right circumstances, any one of us could become depressed.

INFLUENCING FACTORS

Researchers have a long way to go before they understand why people become depressed. Often there is more than one cause, and having a problem that makes you prone to depression does not mean you will develop the condition.

GENES

Genes are important in depression but there are many genes involved and no one knows exactly how they work. There is certainly no evidence of straightforward inheritance for most forms of depression. You will not definitely develop depression because your mother, father, sister or brother has, but your risk will be increased. You will be at highest risk if you have an identical twin who has developed depression.

It is difficult to put figures on this risk because the importance of genes is different for different types of depression. Genetic factors are more important in severe than in mild depression, and more important in young people who get depressed than in older people who get depressed. Genes are most important in the minority of people who have periods when their moods are high and periods when their moods are low – manic depression.

Even if there is a history of depression in the family, there will usually need to be some sort of stressful life event to trigger it.

PERSONALITY

No single type of personality predisposes people to depression. However, those who are obsessional, dogmatic, rigid and who hide their feelings may be more at risk, as may those who get anxious easily. People who have repeated and sustained up and down moods are more likely to develop manic–depressive illness. However, the vast majority of people who have depression do not have any of these personality types.

FAMILY ENVIRONMENT

Certain kinds of traumatic events in a person's childhood are thought to increase the likelihood of depression.

Factors That May Make You Prone to Depression

- Genes
- Personality
- Family environment
- Gender
- Thinking patterns
- Having little control of your destiny
- Stress and life events
- Physical illness
- Lack of daylight

23

Losing a parent in childhood There is some evidence that people who lose their mother when they are young have an increased risk of depression. Suffering that sort of loss might scar you psychologically and make you more susceptible to depression but, on the other hand, it might make you more resilient instead. It may be the psychological, social and financial consequences of losing a parent, rather than the loss itself, that are more important.

Type of parenting Some psychologists claim that demanding, critical parents who take any success for granted, but are harsh on any kind of failure, may make their children more prone to depression in the future. Psychotherapists have suggested that people who have little maternal affection when they are young are at risk of depression in later life, but there is no scientific proof.

Physical or sexual abuse in childhood There is some evidence that physical or sexual abuse can make people prone to severe depression in later life. Studies have shown that up to half of the people who see a psychiatrist have had some kind of unwanted sexual attention during early adolescence or childhood. People who have been abused generally remember the abuse, but some people first remember childhood abuse when they are depressed and are having psychotherapy. There is some disagreement between specialists as to whether these memories are always real. Some argue that, on rare occasions, psychotherapists who believe that sexual abuse is the cause of their patient's problem can make the patient report things that never actually happened by suggesting to him or her that they did. This is known as false memory syndrome.

GENDER

Women are twice as likely to be diagnosed as being depressed as men. This does not necessarily mean women are more prone to depression. It may be that women are more likely to admit to depression than men, or that doctors are more likely to recognise depression in women.

There are, however, social pressures on women that lead to depression that men are less likely to encounter – such as being alone at home with small children. There are also hormonal changes throughout the menstrual cycle, and related to pregnancy and childbirth and to the menopause, that may make women more prone to become depressed or trigger off a bout of depressive illness (for more on this, see p.73).

THINKING PATTERNS

In 1967 an American psychiatrist, Aaron Beck, described patterns of thinking that are common in depression and that he thought made people prone to depression. In short, he believed that people who are very negative about themselves are more likely to suffer from depression.

Most of us have an optimistic way of thinking that keeps us moderately cheerful most of the time. We tend to belittle our failures and make the most of our successes. For example, if you spill a drink in a crowded pub you may say the glasses were overfilled or someone pushed you – it was not your fault. Of course, if you get through the mass of people without spilling a drop you may be unlikely to say the glasses were under-filled or everyone else was careful not to push you. You may claim it as a feat of skill. Some people who are prone to depression think the other way around. They tend to belittle their successes and dwell on their failures.

There is evidence that people think like this when they are depressed, but there is no good evidence they think like this before they get depressed. The importance of this theory is that it has led to cognitive therapy, an exciting new treatment for depression (see p.54).

LACKING CONTROL OVER YOUR DESTINY

FEELING DEPENDENT
A long illness that saps our energy, or a disability that reduces our control over our own lives, can lead to depression.

Some specialists believe that people placed for a long time in a situation over which they have no power and from which they cannot escape are prone to develop depression. The idea came from experiments with dogs performed by a psychologist. He found that the dogs became demoralised, passive and ate less if they were put in experimental conditions where they were given mild punishment for no apparent reason and consequently had no way of controlling the punishment. He called this 'learned helplessness'. Other specialists believe that it is difficult to equate the actions of dogs with those of humans, and it is very difficult to say whether dogs ever get depressed. However, rates of depression are high in those bed-bound or wheelchair-bound patients who rely on nurses for everything.

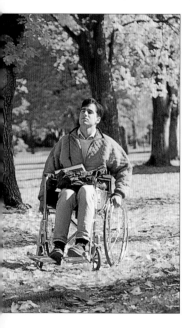

LONG-TERM DISABLING ILLNESSES

Discomfort, disability, dependency and insecurity can make it more likely that a person will become depressed. Most of us prefer to be independent and like to meet people. Being forced into a position where they are relatively helpless may be one way in which severely ill people become prone to depression; or it may be that the energy needed to fight off depression is sapped by long-term illnesses. Worries over financial insecurity may also be important.

TRIGGERING DEPRESSION

Both long-standing and current difficulties may play a part in someone becoming depressed. The experiences that trigger depression are usually losses of some kind – such as losing your job, the death of someone you love (see p.81) or the loss of a partner through divorce – but physical illness can also act as a trigger.

STRESS AND LIFE EVENTS

Stress can lead to depression whether it comes in the form of a sudden, overwhelming event or as long-term stress. Depression is six times more common in the six months after a markedly stressful life event. Stress can make you more prone to developing depression or can trigger it off.

Life events such as loss of a partner or loss of a job may be the final straw if you have long-term difficulties such as housing,-marriage-and/or work problems. The long-term problems magnify the effect of the short-term problem. Experiences that act as triggers may also be losses of a more subtle kind, such as loss of face or the loss of self-esteem through a destructive relationship.

Top 10 Stressful Life Events

- Death of a spouse
- Divorce
- Marital separation
- Prison term
- Death of a close friend
- Injury or illness
- Marriage
- Losing your job
- Marital reconciliation
- Retirement

Only one in 10 of such 'loss events' leads to depression and there are many other experiences in life that sometimes trigger depression but do not involve loss of any kind. We all have our own psychological ways of reacting to stress and it is hard to predict how we will react to particular circumstances.

PHYSICAL ILLNESS

Physical illness can set off depression. The shock of finding out that you have a serious illness can lead to loss of confidence and self-esteem, and so to depression. But the reasons are complex: for instance, depression is quite common after a heart attack, possibly because people feel they had a near miss and it makes them face their own mortality, or perhaps because they become suddenly disabled. In older people physical illness is one of the most common causes of depression.

Illnesses Linked with Depression

- Acromegaly
- Addison's disease
- Alcohol (through direct effects on the brain and consequences for health and social relationships)
- Brain abscess
- Brain haemorrhage
- Brain tumours
- Chronic fatigue syndrome
- Cushing's disease
- Dementia
- Diabetes
- Encephalitis
- Head injuries
- Heart problems
- Hyperparathyroidism
- Hypopituitarism
- Hypothyroidism
- Multiple sclerosis
- Parkinson's disease
- Tuberculosis
- Meningitis
- Vitamin deficiency
- Viral illnesses (including 'flu and glandular fever)
- Water balance problems (such as low salt, high calcium or low calcium in your body)

Some illnesses can cause depression because of the way they affect the body. Depression can accompany Parkinson's disease and multiple sclerosis partly because of their effects on the brain. Illnesses that affect your hormones can cause depression. There is also a link with viral illnesses: an epidemic of influenza is often followed by an epidemic of depression, and many of us will know someone who has become depressed after a bout of glandular fever. How a virus causes depression is not clear, but one theory is that viruses use up the body's supplies of vitamins, so weakening it.

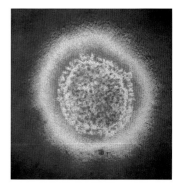

INFLUENZA VIRUS
Various kinds of viral infection, including 'flu and glandular fever, can produce depression, possibly because they weaken the body.

MEDICINES AND DRUGS

Some prescription medications can cause depression, but you should not stop taking any of the medicines in the list on the right without consulting your doctor. These drugs do not always cause depression and you may have another reason for being depressed. Stopping the medication you are taking can be more dangerous than depression.

Non-prescription drugs can also lead to depression. Alcohol has direct effects on the brain and can make you feel depressed. Alcoholism can also cause depression because of the negative effect it has on your life. Similarly, recreational drugs can cause depression through direct effects and the impact they have on your lifestyle.

Medicines That May Cause Depression

- Anti-epilepsy tablets
- Anti-high blood pressure drugs
- Anti-parkinsonian drugs
- Contraceptive pill (combined contraceptive pill and possibly progestogen-only pill)
- Digitalis
- Diuretics
- Major tranquillisers
- Steroid therapy (for asthma, arthritis, etc.)

LACK OF DAYLIGHT

Most of us feel better in the sun than on overcast days and prefer the summer to the winter, but this takes an extreme form in some individuals. They are fine in summer but become depressed as the days grow shorter at the onset of winter. They are said to suffer from seasonal affective disorder (SAD).

SAD may be related to the levels of a hormone called melatonin, which is released from the pineal gland in the brain. Its release is sensitive to light; more is released when it is dark. Light therapy is sometimes very effective in getting rid of the symptoms of SAD. Four hours of bright light a day from a special lamp can lift depression within about a week.

KEY POINTS

- There are many possible reasons for depression.
- Some physical illnesses and some medications can cause depression.
- Usually there are a number of causes for any person's depressive illness.

Types of depression

Your feelings of depression are highly personal, but your doctor, counsellor or another professional can distinguish between broad types of the illness by cause, symptoms and duration.

CLASSIFYING DEPRESSION

Throughout this book you will find that the terms mild, moderate and severe are used to describe the three broad categories of depression that have clear distinguishing characteristics.

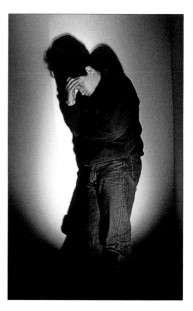

MILD DEPRESSION

In mild depression the low mood may come and go and the illness often starts after a specific stressful event. The person may have feelings of anxiety as well as feeling low. Lifestyle changes are often all that are needed to lift this kind of depression.

MODERATE DEPRESSION

In moderate depression the low mood is persistent and the person manifests physical symptoms in addition, although these symptoms will vary from person to person. Changes in lifestyle alone are unlikely to work and medical help is needed.

FEELING LOW
A low mood that comes and goes suggests mild depression, which may respond to lifestyle changes. If it persists and you have physical symptoms of depression then you should seek medical help.

31

SEVERE

Severe depression is a life-threatening illness in which symptoms are intense. The person will experience physical symptoms, delusions and hallucinations, and it is important that they see a doctor as soon as possible.

— OTHER TERMS FOR DEPRESSION —

Other terms in common use among the medical profession to describe types of depression include:

REACTIVE DEPRESSION

This term is used in two ways by doctors. In the first, reactive is used to describe a depression that is caused by a stressful event – such as losing your job – and does not usually last long. It could be described as a short-lived exaggeration of a normal response to adversity. Counselling, family support, stress management and practical steps may be all that are needed to treat it.

However, a stressful event can trigger more severe depression and people who are prone to depression can have stressful life events after their illness starts. If this happens, it is difficult to pinpoint exactly whether the depression is truly a reaction to stress.

Reactive is also used to describe a depression in which a person can still react to and enjoy social situations.

ENDOGENOUS DEPRESSION

Endogenous depression comes on for no reason; it is usually intense and the person is likely to have physical symptoms of depression, such as loss of appetite and weight, early morning wakening, mood worse in the morning and loss of interest in sex. It will usually only get better with treatment.

The trouble with using this particular way of defining depression is that the same symptoms can be triggered in some people by stressful events. Further-more, just because you cannot put your finger on any particular stress-ful event that set the depression off, it does not mean that there was not one.

NEUROTIC DEPRESSION

This term is used to describe a mild form of depression in which the person has good and bad days. He or she tends to feel more depressed in the evenings. With this kind of depression, you may well experience difficulty getting off to sleep and have interrupted sleep but no early morning wakening. Some people sleep excessively, and some find that they are more irritable than usual.

LOSING INTEREST
Endogenous depression is usually intense and will often result in a diminished sex drive. Treatment is generally necessary.

Neurotic can be used as a derogatory term, so the description neurotic depression is not used much these days and, in any case, it is really just another name for mild depression.

PSYCHOTIC DEPRESSION

Psychotic depression is severe, and people who are suffering from it will experience physical symptoms and may lose touch with reality. They may have delusions and/or hallucinations. People with psychotic depression always need medical treatment.

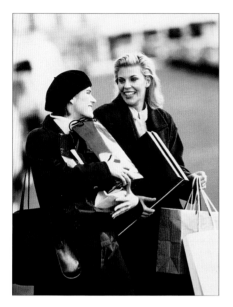

POOR JUDGEMENT
Whilst in the high mood of bipolar depression, sufferers may indulge in extravagant spending, deluded into thinking they can afford it.

BIPOLAR DEPRESSION

Bipolar depression is another name for manic–depressive illness. People who have a manic–depressive illness have sustained high moods and periods of sustained low moods that can range from mild to severe depression. When a person with this illness is in one of the high moods (manic), they are likely to feel elated, need less sleep or food than usual and experience a general feeling of well-being. They have excessive amounts of energy, speak very quickly and feel as if thoughts are racing in their head. Their judgement is likely to be poor and they may also experience hallucinations and delusions, but these are the opposite to those in psychotic depression – their content is much more positive. Some people believe that they know the Royal Family or that they are VIPs when they are not, others believe that they are rich or have special powers. High moods can be as destructive as low ones, and sometimes the lack of sound judgement and delusions can lead to financial trouble as a result of impulse buying – in some cases a yacht or a wildly expensive house.

UNIPOLAR DEPRESSION

Unipolar depression is a term that is used to describe the kind of depression experienced by the vast majority of people and means that they have only low moods, not high ones as well.

AGITATED DEPRESSION

Agitated depression is actually a description of the symptoms of this particular type of depression, in which the individual is anxious, worried and restless.

RETARDED DEPRESSION

Retarded depression is again a description of symptoms and refers to the kind of depression in which both mental and physical processes are slowed down and the person often finds it difficult to concentrate. When the illness is very severe, some people find it impossible to move, speak or eat, and there is a risk that they might starve.

DYSTHYMIA

This term refers to mild depression that is persistent. Although it may come and go, doctors will make this diagnosis if the illness has gone on for more than two months in a two-year period. The main symptoms are indecision and low self-esteem. Psychotherapy may work better than drug treatment.

MASKED, OR SMILING, DEPRESSION

People with masked depression say they do not feel depressed, even though they have a number of other symptoms that point to depression. They may be investigated for physical illnesses before the diagnosis is made. Physical symptoms, such as chest pain or sleep problems, get better when the person is given anti-depressant treatment.

ORGANIC DEPRESSION

This is the name given to a kind of depression that is caused by a physical illness or medication.

BRIEF RECURRENT DEPRESSION

This term is used to refer to a recently recognised illness in which serious depression comes on and lasts for only a few days at a time.

SEASONAL AFFECTIVE DISORDER (SAD)

This term was originally used to mean any depressive illness that came on regularly at a certain time of year – say because of increased demands at work. It is now used for a specific type of depression that results from decreasing levels of daylight as winter approaches and days get shorter. People with SAD may experience craving for carbohydrate and/or chocolate and an increased need for sleep during the winter months.

KEY POINTS

- There are many types of depression.
- Mild depression may not need drug treatment, but moderate and severe depression often do.
- Depression may be persistent or come and go and may be associated with other symptoms.

Helping yourself

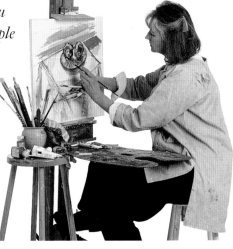

When your depression is mild, you may well be able to benefit from simple self-help measures, but when your condition is more severe they should be used as part of a plan discussed with your doctor or therapist. They may help to stave off depression as well as to treat it and promote recovery.

This chapter contains a range of such measures, but do not try to do everything at once. Consider which of them could make a difference to you and then have a go.

So Much You Can Do
Many kinds of change in your life can leave you with time on your hands, and an absorbing pastime can help to fend off depression.

PREPARING FOR DIFFICULTIES

People often become depressed following a loss of some kind, but it may be possible to prepare yourself when you know you are going to have to face up to a change. The sort of predictable things that can trigger depression include loss of social support when a person goes to university, loss of freedom or work status when a woman takes maternity leave and loss of work routine and social contact for some people when they retire. Not surprisingly, rates of depression are high at these times. There are two ways to decrease the stress of predictable losses: the first is by being open and acknowledging that there may be a problem; the second is by preparing for the change. If you acknowledge your feelings you will feel better. If you are ambivalent about the change in your life, talk it through with a friend – let other people know your concerns and they may be able to support you. Saying how you feel may change the way people treat you: for example, if you are retiring, they may stop telling you that you should be happy at not having to work any more, they may spend more time with you or expect less of you while you are adjusting to your new situation.

Good preparation for any change is helpful; reading about it, or talking to people who have gone through a similar experience, will be useful. Taking common-sense measures to decrease the stress and trying to arrange your first few days or weeks in advance may help the transition. For instance, if you are going to university, you may find that there are people you know there whom you could arrange to meet up with, or you could practise cooking some simple meals before you go so that you have one less problem to fret about.

The early weeks of retirement can be planned so that there is social support and you have something to do. Many women find support groups, such as the National Childbirth Trust, invaluable after they have had a baby.

GET AWAY FROM IT ALL
It does not have to be on a tropical beach, but a holiday – even a short one – may raise your spirits and give you a better perspective.

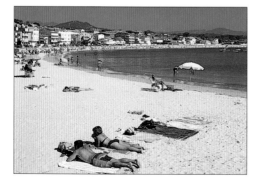

TAKE A BREAK

If you are feeling down or you feel that everything is getting on top of you, take a break, even if you can only manage a day or a night away. Better still, take a proper holiday if you can. It is not running away and you will only get a little behind in your work. You will probably find that you can think through your problems better if you are away from them, and you may work much better when you get back. A break may give you the rest you need to attack your problems and the distance to put them in proper perspective. If you find that you cannot enjoy a few days away, this is a sign that you need professional help.

TALK THINGS OVER

You will find that if you talk problems over with your partner, a friend or a family member, you will feel better. It not only decreases the burden on you, but just talking through things may help you find a solution. You may discover that your friends have their own ideas about what you should do, and they may think of solutions that have not occurred to you. They may have gone through the same kind of difficulties that you are experiencing and so be able to give you insights into your problems.

People often feel better after they have had a good cry. The open acknowledgement of your problems is often the starting point for working out solutions.

Many people who are depressed cut themselves off and think they are a burden to other people. In fact, this just makes you more depressed, so do try instead to choose a friend who will be sympathetic and willing to listen to you and help you through a difficult time. Everyone needs help at some time.

CHANGE YOUR LIFESTYLE

See whether you can identify and change aspects of your life that may have brought on the depression. You may need help to do this but it is not as impractical as it seems.

Somebody else will usually have gone through a similar problem before, and there may be a way you can solve the problem too. If you are worried about an illness you should discuss this with your doctor; things may not be as bad as they seem. If it is a social or legal problem you could visit a Citizens Advice Bureau for help.

GET IN TOUCH WITH A GROUP

There are many ways in which other people can help, and joining a group of some kind can be a real support. Some organisations that may help are listed in the section starting on p.91. Your GP should have information about what is available in your area. If you need help urgently and do not want to see your GP then call the Samaritans. They offer telephone and face-to-face counselling.

There are a number of other organisations that offer more specialised help – for example, if your relationship is the cause of your depression, you could contact Relate (formerly the Marriage Guidance Council) who will see you with your partner or alone. If you need help with bereavement, CRUSE may help. These organisations are also listed in the 'Useful addresses' section.

LOOK AFTER YOURSELF

If you are feeling depressed keeping occupied often helps. Taking up a new activity or hobby at an evening class or at the weekend is one idea. Getting out of the house and meeting people will do you good because it breaks the vicious circle of loneliness and spending too much time mulling over your problems.

Make a conscious effort to do what you like doing – listening to a record, going shopping, having a massage, going to a concert or a film. Little things can make a big difference. Exercise can boost your well-being too. It does not just make you feel better psychologically, it also gets you out of the house and makes you fitter. Exercise does not have to be Lycra-style aerobics. Going for a good walk or a swim will do just as well. Active pastimes such as bowling are a good way of getting out and doing something. If you have not done any exercise for a while, you should be careful and start slowly.

Even if you do not have much of an appetite make sure that you eat regularly, and if you cannot face a meal go for balanced snacks instead. If you do not eat properly you will not have the physical strength to get better and may start descending into the vicious circle of worse and worse depression. If you really cannot face eating properly, or preparing a meal, soluble powders, such as Complan, can be bought from pharmacies and supermarkets without a prescription. They contain a whole day's nourishment that is taken in a liquid form and they are easy to prepare.

Remember that alcohol will not sort out your problems. It will make you feel more depressed and could become a habit that ruins your life. Alcohol decreases inhibitions and may lead to suicidal impulses taking over. You should also be careful about drinking alcohol if you are taking antidepressants.

NOT A SOLUTION
Alcohol will not solve your depression – it is far more likely to make matters worse in other areas of your life, such as health and relationships.

Sleeping problems are very common and depressed people are especially prone to insomnia. In addition, lack of sleep makes it more difficult to summon up the energy to fight depression. If your depression is moderate or severe, self-help may not be enough to cure any sleeping problems and you may require medication to sort out your insomnia.

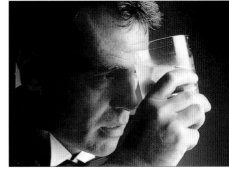

STRESS MANAGEMENT

Reducing the amount of stress in your life is one of the most positive steps you can take to lessen the symptoms and severity of your depression. There are many ways in which to relieve stress, but learning how to relax properly is an easy and beneficial first step.

RELAXATION

Learning how to relax is easier said than done and is something that many of us need help to do. Fortunately, there are many ways of relieving tension and one of them will work for you.

One thing that many relaxation techniques have in common is that they teach you to recognise when your muscles are tense and how to relieve that tension. You can learn this technique by going to a relaxation group, by buying relaxation tapes or by reading about it. Your GP may have a relaxation group or relaxation trainer at the surgery. This is often a good place to start and after a couple of sessions you will probably be able to relax properly yourself at home.

There are also more elaborate methods of relaxation, such as meditation, and of teaching you to know when you are tense, for example using a technique called biofeedback.

Biofeedback relaxation This method is aided by a machine that monitors either muscle responses or electrical activity in the skin. When you are feeling more tense, electrical activity in the skin and muscle increases and this causes the machine to produce a signal – either a high-pitched whistle or a light that comes on. When you relax the sound gets lower in frequency or the light goes off – so you learn when to relax your muscles.

How to Get a Good Night's Sleep

Prolonged bouts of insomnia can be very stressful and will make your depression much more difficult to cope with. Listed below are some useful tips to help you get a good night's sleep.

- Get up earlier in the morning to see if this helps.
- Take some exercise during the day.
- Do not take naps.
- Do not exercise just before bed – it can make it difficult to sleep.
- Do not have a heavy meal late at night as you could feel uncomfortable – but do not go to bed hungry. Do not drink coffee, tea or cola in the evening.
- Get your mind off your problems by reading a book before trying to sleep.
- Go to bed at a regular time so that your body sets up a natural rhythm.
- Do not drink alcohol to help you sleep – it may not work and you may not be able to break the habit.
- Make sure your bed is comfortable.
- Have a warm milky drink last thing before going to bed.
- Adjust the heating and ventilation so that the room is not too hot or too cold.
- Do not smoke before you go to sleep – nicotine is a stimulant.
- Sexual intercourse before you go to sleep can help you wind down.
- Do relaxation exercises before you try to go to sleep.
- Remember – if you cannot get off to sleep for half an hour or if you wake up at night and can't get back to sleep, get up and read a book or watch television. Lying there worrying will not do you any good – it could make things worse!

Autogenic training This is a series of simple mental exercises in which the patient is encouraged to enter a state of passive concentration – it is a form of meditation that can reduce stress and make individuals more relaxed. You will usually need professional help for these exercises, and many of the techniques involved in autogenic training are no more effective than simple relaxation training.

MASSAGE

Massage can be done by yourself, your partner or a professional. There are plenty of devices that can be bought to help you massage yourself, but it is usually best to get someone else to do it. You may be able to talk over your problems at the same time.

Specialist types of massage are all good for stress.

Shiatsu This is a Japanese massage technique based upon traditional Chinese medical theory. Our vital life force, or *Qi*, is believed to flow through our bodies in certain pathways or meridians. If it gets blocked, or there is an imbalance, disease occurs. In Shiatsu massage, pressure points are manipulated to unblock or balance the flow of *Qi* energy.

HEALING HANDS
Shiatsu massage works on specific pressure points of the body to unblock the flow of Qi energy.

Reflexology This is another ancient art of massage. Different areas on the foot are thought to be linked to certain body systems. Manipulation and massage of these areas are thought to put right problems that you have in the particular body system.

Aromatherapy This uses the scents of plant oils and essential oils to aid psychological well-being.

PET THERAPY

Some people who are prone to recurrent depression find it is therapeutic to get a dog or a cat. They are cuddly, reliable and responsive and may decrease your stress level. However, being given a pet when you are depressed will not necessarily make you better. Apart from the fact that caring for a pet requires a lot of time and effort, it takes time to build up a relationship.

Relaxation Exercise

*This is a simple method for relaxing. It only takes 20 minutes maximum.
You can do it in bed, lying on the floor or sitting in a comfortable chair. Just make sure any chair
you use supports your neck. You may want to try it in the evening first time around – some
people feel so relaxed they fall asleep. Once you've got the hang of it you will be able
to do it anywhere without dropping off, unless you want to.*

1. Let your whole body go limp. Try to feel as heavy on the bed or in the chair as possible. Let the bed or the chair take your weight. Feel heavy, like a sack of potatoes.

2. Put your arms by your side and let them flop down. Let your legs go all floppy as well. Let your shoulders drop. Relax all parts of your body from the top down. Feel heavy on the bed or chair.

3. If you have not done relaxation exercises before, you will need to teach yourself how to relax your muscles. Tense the muscle in your upper leg harder and harder until you cannot tense it any more. Now release it. You will feel the difference between tension and relaxation. Do the same from the top of your body to your toes. Start with your face – screw your face up, clench your teeth and then release. Then make your neck muscles tense, then release. Shrug your shoulders so they nearly touch your ears, then let them drop. Tense and release your arms, chest, stomach, backside, legs, feet and toes, one by one.

4. You will find that your muscles feel less tense than they did when you started. Remember what they feel like. Once you have the hang of it you will not need to tense your muscles before you relax them.

5. When you feel relaxed and limp – slow your breathing down bit by bit, making it slow and even. Concentrate only on your breathing. Make inhaling and exhaling the same length, long and slow. Stop if you feel light-headed. After 20 minutes you will feel much better than when you started. You will feel calmer and more rested.

COMPLEMENTARY MEDICINE

Many people with depression turn to alternative forms of therapy, and some of these prove effective, but it may be best to check with your GP first.

HOMEOPATHY

Homeopathy is a form of medicine built on the principle that like heals like, and that very small quantities of a substance are needed to promote healing. For instance, a nettle extract may be prescribed for a skin rash, but this nettle extract will be so dilute that very little in the way of nettle remains. Despite this, the nettle extract is thought to promote the body's own immune system. Before you consider going to see a homeopath of your own accord, talk it over with your doctor first. Some GPs are trained homeopaths and there are homeopathic NHS hospitals. Your doctor can advise you whether going to a homeopath with your particular depression is a good idea, and he or she may know a good local practitioner.

ACUPUNCTURE

Acupuncture works on the same principles of *Qi* as Shiatsu; however, rather than massage, fine needles are inserted in points on the meridians to help balance *Qi*. Acupuncture is increasingly being used in the UK and there are a number of doctors trained in acupuncture as well as in conventional Western medicine. Its effectiveness in treating depression is still a matter for debate.

HYPNOSIS

Hypnosis can be used to aid relaxation but is not a treatment for depression. In hypnosis you are not asleep

– you enter a trance and the hypnotist attempts to help you to manipulate your subconscious mind.

Some types of hypnosis have been used to stop people feeling anxious, but there is little good evidence for them working in depression.

KEY POINTS

- Self-help can be part of a plan agreed with your GP.

- Do not try to change everything at one time.

- Once you are well, self-help techniques may stave off depression in the future.

Treating depression

If self-help does not work, or if your depression is severe from the outset, you should see your GP. He or she knows about depression and will listen to you, may know you and your medical history and can make sure that there are no physical problems that are causing the depression.

FIRST PORT OF CALL
Your GP is trained to help you and will understand your problem. If further help is needed, he or she will know what specialist help is available locally.

Your GP can also arrange investigations or start treatment, will be there to offer you support, can sign you off work if necessary, can refer you to a specialist and will know other therapies available in your area.

Whilst your GP should be the first port of call if you need help, if there is an emergency you can call the Samaritans or visit your local accident and emergency department. There, you will be assessed by a doctor and a psychiatrist can be called if necessary. In some areas hospitals have emergency psychiatric clinics that you can just walk into; in other areas there is a crisis intervention team who will see you at home.

Each of these services is used to dealing with people who are depressed and will offer high-quality treatment. No one will think that your problems are trivial or stupid. They will be eager to help – that is what they are there for.

There are three types of treatment for depression – psychological treatment, drug treatment and physical treatment. The first two may be available through your GP; the last is only available from specialists and only used in very severe depression.

PSYCHOLOGICAL THERAPIES

Psychological therapies are the most popular type of treatment for depression, partly because they do not involve taking tablets and partly because they make intuitive sense. It seems right to sit down and talk about things if they are getting on top of us. It also seems right to try to get to the bottom of why we feel the way we do when depression comes on for no reason.

However, you may be too depressed to be able to think clearly and may be too tired to start psychotherapy. All psychological therapies take a lot of time and commitment. They are not an easy option. They take a lot of energy. You may need to lift your depression with antidepressant medication before you consider psychological treatment. You should see your doctor to discuss what is available in your area.

There are many different types of psychological therapy and they are based on different theories. They are most easily split into brief therapies, which last at most six months, long-term therapies, which last longer, and counselling. Brief therapies usually consist of four to 20 weekly sessions, each lasting up to an hour. In long-term therapies there are usually over 50 sessions; they are often weekly but they can be five times a week.

What Happens when You Visit Your GP?

If you think you are suffering from depression, your GP is the first person to consult. He or she will be able to offer experienced help.

- Your GP will discuss your problems and make sure that they are not the result of a physical illness.

- Your GP will decide how severe your depression is.

- If you have mild depression, you may not be prescribed medication. You will be given advice, may be offered psychotherapy or counselling and your GP will see you again to make sure things get better.

- If you have moderate depression, your GP may offer you antidepressants and may refer you for psychotherapy or counselling.

- If you do not want to take antidepressants your GP will monitor your progress – you should strongly consider taking the tablets if your GP thinks you need them.

- If you have severe depression your GP may treat you but may refer you to a psychiatrist. This will depend on your symptoms.

- Your GP will want to see you a week or two after starting antidepressants. This is to make sure that you do not have side-effects and you can continue to take the tablets.

- If you cannot tolerate the drugs they can be changed – so tell your GP if you have problems.

- The drugs work gradually; sleep and tiredness improve first – depressed mood often last.

- You will need to see your GP regularly to get more tablets and to make sure things are going well.

What Happens when You Visit Your GP? (cont'd)

- After six weeks you should feel much better.

- Even though you feel much better you should continue to take your tablets for another six months or so. After this you will come off them slowly, not all in one go.

- If you are not better, your GP may increase the dose and see you again in three weeks.

- If you are better after this time, your GP will keep you on the tablets for at least six months before you come off them slowly.

- If you are still not better, most GPs will then refer you to a psychiatrist.

- The psychiatrist will assess you again to make sure that nothing else is causing the depression. If not, you may be offered a different type of medication.

- If you are not better in a month, the psychiatrist will consider offering a different drug, a combination of drugs or admitting you to hospital for investigation and assessment.

- If nothing else works and you are very depressed you may be offered ECT.

- If you are severely depressed from the outset – deluded, suicidal or not eating and drinking – your GP may refer you straight to a psychiatrist. You may be offered admission to hospital so that treatment can be started in a safe environment.

Treating Different Types of Depression

Depending upon whether your GP or another specialist judges your depression to be mild, moderate or severe, different kinds of treatment will be recommended.

MILD DEPRESSION

Self-help, lifestyle changes and psychotherapy often work. Medication may not work at all. However, new research has shown that if you have had mild depression for years a combination of antidepressants and psychotherapy can lead to an improvement.

MODERATE DEPRESSION

Either medication or psychotherapy can work here depending on your symptoms. Some GPs believe that both are required. If you have early morning wakening, depression worse in the morning, loss of appetite or weight and loss of interest in things that you used to enjoy, antidepressants will work well. If you would prefer psychotherapy, you need to be monitored regularly by your doctor. If things get worse, you should reconsider starting medication.

SEVERE DEPRESSION

Most people with severe depression are too ill to benefit from psychotherapy and need to take antidepressants. People who are actively suicidal need urgent help and to be in a safe place. If the depression is characterised by delusions and hallucinations, an antidepressant may be combined with a special drug, an antipsychotic, which will specifically treat these.

RECURRENT DEPRESSION

If you have been depressed before, you should use the treatment that worked last time because it will do so again. Once you are well you should discuss long-term treatment with your doctor – lithium or a low dose of antidepressant can help stave off another attack.

MANIC–DEPRESSIVE ILLNESS

Depression can be treated with antidepressants, but your doctor will want to monitor your treatment carefully because, in a few people with up and down moods, antidepressants can lead to a high mood. In the long term, other medications that act as mood stabilisers – such as lithium or carbamazepine – may be more suitable.

Brief therapies usually deal with problems in the here and now, whereas long-term therapies delve into the past to try to discover why you are the way you are. Counselling lasts for a variable time, from one session onwards. It does not aim to change deep-rooted problems or treat your depression, but it may help get rid of some of the problems that are causing you to be depressed.

BRIEF THERAPIES

Many brief therapies are available on the NHS and your GP or a psychiatrist may suggest you try one of these. The possibilities include cognitive therapy, behaviour therapy, cognitive–behaviour therapy and cognitive analytical therapy, all of which have been used in depression. Which kind of therapy you are offered may depend on what is available locally.

A good therapist is probably as important as the type of therapy on offer. Your therapist may be a doctor, a nurse, a psychologist, an occupational thera-pist or a social worker. If you have NHS psycho-therapy it is likely that it will be supervised by a consultant psychotherapist to make sure that things go well. There are several kinds of brief therapy, each with its own strengths.

Cognitive therapy This therapy works specifically on depressive thinking patterns. You will be asked to record your negative thoughts and look at the way you think. You will then be helped to challenge thoughts that are unrealistically negative. Over 10–20 weekly sessions, the therapist tries to help you to stop thinking in a depressed way. This has been shown to work in even moderately severe depression. It can have benefits that last longer than medication alone. It can be used in combination with antidepressants. If you suffer from depression you should consider cognitive therapy seriously.

For instance, our secretary Carrie (see p.13) would be asked to work through her belief that she is a failure and present evidence for and against it. She would be helped to see that there are other ways of looking at the problem and that she does not have to be so hard on herself. She would be helped to think in a more balanced way. Perhaps she is not the best secretary in the world but she is a good secretary, and even good secretaries make mistakes from time to time.

Behaviour therapy This treatment differs from cognitive therapy in that it focuses on what we do rather than what we think. Rather than trying to make you think less depressed, it makes you act less depressed. A behaviour modification programme may try to get you sleeping well, looking after yourself better and eating more sensibly. It stops you 'giving up'. Some people find this a first step back to recovery.

In Carrie's case, all of these may be employed to make sure she does not slip into a more severe depression. She would be encouraged to look after herself, develop good sleep and eating habits and make sure she does not get into a depressive downward spiral.

Cognitive–behaviour therapy This uses elements of cognitive therapy and behaviour therapy to good effect in depression. It is a newer therapy, but it is being used more and more.

Cognitive analytical therapy This is another new therapy. It uses cognitive and behavioural techniques, but also looks into your past to give you an idea where your ways of thinking come from. It is one of the few brief therapies that gives reasons for your problems.

If Carrie talked about her past it may have become clear that her parents were very critical. Her feelings of inferiority may have come from the way she was undermined as a child. If Carrie could realise that the way she felt was because of circumstances and her childhood she may find it easier to accept herself for what she is and be less self-critical, dissatisfied and depressed as a result.

LONG-TERM THERAPY

There are many different types of long-term therapy, all based on different theories. They may be available on the NHS, but there are usually long waiting lists. Long-term therapies try to deal with the deep-rooted causes of depression. They are not a quick form of treatment. Their aim is to sort out long-standing problems, and they may not make you feel any less depressed in the short term.

Psychoanalysis Psychoanalysts believe that our difficulties are caused by problems from the past that we have not dealt with. We may have denied them, ignored them or tried to forget them, but they are still in the backs of our minds. They stay there and fester and come back to us when we are under stress or weakened in some way. They can also weaken us. Such a problem could be the loss of a parent when we were young, at which time there was no proper grieving process and feelings were just covered up.

Long-term psychotherapy is said to work by helping these bad feelings come to the surface and into the consciousness. The aim is to disarm the feelings and to stop them causing problems.

SIGMUND FREUD
The founding father of psychoanalysis, Freud believed that psychological illnesses stem from unresolved problems in our past.

If you are thinking of having this sort of therapy, you should discuss it with your GP. There is a bewildering choice of people who offer psychotherapy and some are poorly trained practitioners.

Counselling Counsellors try to help you solve problems. They will not give advice, but they will help you to make decisions. Many counsellors are trained but some are not, so it is a good idea to ask your GP for a recommendation. You may even find that your GP has a counsellor in his or her surgery.

ANTIDEPRESSANT MEDICATION

Antidepressant tablets are a very effective treatment for depression. When they are taken as prescribed they should improve symptoms within two weeks, although it can often take six weeks for the full benefit to be felt. You should normally continue taking antidepressant tablets for at least six months after the depression has lifted, to make sure that it does not return, and then gradually stop the treatment. These drugs work well for moderate and severe depression.

Many people think they will become addicted to, or dependent on, antidepressants, but this will not happen. Antidepressants are not like Valium (diazepam) and are not addictive. They only work if you are depressed and will not work if you are not. They do not give you a high. There is a black market trade in nearly all drugs that give you a high and can be addictive – there is no black market trade in antidepressants.

However, antidepressants are powerful drugs and some people who stop them suddenly feel peculiar. This is not a sign that you are addicted to, or dependent on, antidepressants, it is just that the body is used to having them around. Once your depression is better, a gradual reduction in dose in the weeks before stopping will ensure that your body resets itself and that there are no symptoms.

HOW DO ANTIDEPRESSANTS WORK?

In depression there are physical changes to the way in which your body works, and antidepressants put things back to normal. As we saw earlier (see p.19), nerve cells in the brain are separated by a small space – the synapse. In order to pass messages to each other, nerve cells release chemicals (neurotransmitters) that leave one nerve cell and cross the space to the next nerve cell – like a baton in a relay race. The message is only passed on if there is enough neurotransmitter in the synapse. After release, the neurotransmitters are broken up or taken back into the brain cell that released them.

The levels of these neurotransmitters are low in depression – it is as if the baton were being dropped. Antidepressants work by increasing the amount of neurotransmitters in the space between the cells – they put the baton back into the hand of the nerve cell.

The amount of neurotransmitter in the synapse can be increased by various drugs, which work in different ways:
● Increasing the amount of neurotransmitter that is made (tryptophan).
● Preventing neurotransmitters being broken down (monoamine oxidase inhibitors or MAOIs).
● Stopping neurotransmitters in the synapse being taken back up into the cells (tricyclics, tricyclic-like compounds, SSRIs).

Over time the body rights itself, the amounts of neurotransmitters naturally produced increase and antidepressants are no longer needed.

How Do Antidepressants Treat Depression

In depression, the levels of neurotransmitters are low. Antidepressant drugs work to increase levels in one of three ways – by increasing the amount of neurotransmitter made, by stopping the breakdown of neurotransmitters or by inhibiting reabsorption.

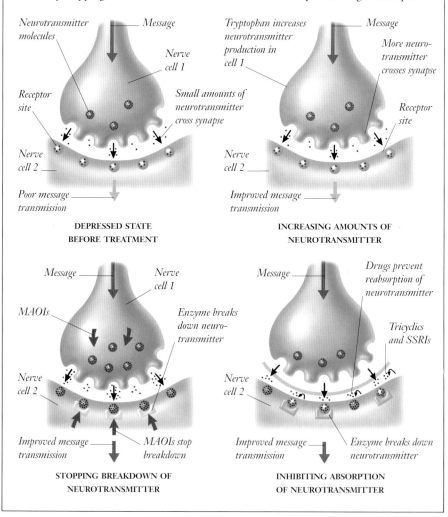

Neurotransmitter molecules — *Message*

Nerve cell 1

Receptor site

Small amounts of neurotransmitter cross synapse

Nerve cell 2

Poor message transmission

**DEPRESSED STATE
BEFORE TREATMENT**

Tryptophan increases neurotransmitter production in cell 1 — *Message*

More neuro-transmitter crosses synapse

Receptor site

Nerve cell 2

Improved message transmission

**INCREASING AMOUNTS OF
NEUROTRANSMITTER**

Message — *Nerve cell 1*

MAOIs

Enzyme breaks down neuro-transmitter

Nerve cell 2

Improved message transmission — *MAOIs stop breakdown*

**STOPPING BREAKDOWN OF
NEUROTRANSMITTER**

Drugs prevent reabsorption of neurotransmitter

Message

Tricyclics and SSRIs

Nerve cell 2

Improved message transmission — *Enzyme breaks down neurotransmitter*

**INHIBITING ABSORPTION
OF NEUROTRANSMITTER**

Who Needs Antidepressants?

If you are mildly depressed you probably do not need this kind of treatment; with moderate depression you probably do and with severe depression you definitely do.

Any medication should be prescribed after a full consultation with your GP or a psychiatrist and as part of an agreed plan that might also include self-help techniques and psychotherapy. If you are having drug treatment this should be discussed with the therapist. If you are hesitant about taking antidepressants, remember that doctors do not prescribe antidepressants to fob patients off. You may find it impossible to work through your problems unless you take them.

Certain symptoms, such as early morning wakening, depression that is worse in the morning, loss of appetite and weight and loss of interest in things you used to enjoy, indicate that your depression is very likely to respond to antidepressants.

The medication may have side-effects. These are at their worst when you start treatment but get better as your body gets used to it. They can be reduced by starting at a low dose and building up, or by changing the drug you are on. Most side-effects are less of a bother than the depression. If the drugs are taken properly, your depression will improve. Antidepressants work best if you take a full dose. Low doses are not as effective, and you may end up with side-effects but no benefit. Try to persevere. There are many different antidepressants available, and they all work. Some are better for one type of depression than another, and different kinds have different side-effects.

After one episode of depression you will be advised to stay on medication for six months to make sure that the depression does not return. If you have had a previous bout of depression you may be advised to stay on medication for longer. Some doctors now advise their patients to stay on medication indefinitely if they have their first bout of depression after the age of 50 because there is a significant risk of a further bout.

TRICYCLIC ANTIDEPRESSANTS

These chemicals are called tricyclics because of their chemical structure – three rings that are linked together, with a side chain (like a tricycle). They increase the amount of neurotransmitter between brain cells by preventing the neurotransmitter from being reabsorbed by the cell that released it. They are very effective in moderate or severe depression in which there are problems with sleeping, appetite, agitation or retardation. They take up to two weeks to start working.

There are many different tricyclic antidepressants. They all work on depression but may have other effects too. For example, some are sedatives that calm you down – others are not.

If you are anxious and agitated your doctor will probably prescribe a sedative antidepressant. However, if you feel slow and tired all the time your doctor will probably opt for one that is less sedative. Some people taking sedative tricyclics feel drowsy during the day. This can be reduced by taking the whole day's dose at night rather than three times a day. This may also make you sleep better. If you drive for a living or use machinery, you should take special care when taking anti-depressants. Discuss this with your doctor.

Tricyclic Antidepressants

SEDATIVE TRICYCLICS:

- Amitriptyline
- Clomipramine
- Dothiepin
- Doxepin
- Trimipramine

STIMULANT TRICYCLIC:

- Protriptyline

NON-SEDATIVE TRICYCLICS:

- Amoxapine
- Desipramine
- Imipramine
- Lofepramine
- Nortriptyline

Tricyclics are powerful drugs and, like all powerful drugs, they can have side-effects, but some of the newer ones, such as lofepramine, have relatively few. Not everyone gets side-effects but, if you do, tell your doctor. They can be reduced by starting the medi-cation at a low level and building up the dose. They can also be reduced by changing the tricyclic that you take.

These antidepressants can interfere with other tablets that you take – even hay fever tablets bought over the counter – so you should consult your doctor and pharmacist before taking anything else. An overdose of tricyclics can be fatal. There should only be a small number of these pills in the house if someone is suicidal.

Some Side-effects of Tricyclics

- Blurring of vision
- Constipation
- In men, difficulty getting an erection and ejaculating
- Difficulty passing water
- Dry mouth
- Effects on the heart (makes it beat fast or irregularly)
- Fits (rare and occur only in people who are prone to them)
- Giddiness on standing
- Excessive sweating
- Tremor of the hands
- Weight gain

TRICYCLIC-LIKE ANTIDEPRESSANTS

There are many drugs that act just like tricyclics but that do not have the three-ring structure and therefore are not called tricyclics. For example:

- Maprotiline has four rings. It should not be taken if you have had epilepsy.
- Mianserin has few side-effects apart from an effect on the bone marrow, but for this reason it tends to be used less often.
- Iprindole can, very rarely, cause liver problems.
- Trazodone has few side-effects, although, in men, it can very rarely cause an erection that does not go away; this is quite painful.
- Viloxazine has fewer side-effects than most tricyclics.

● Mirtazapine is an effective antidepressant that can cause blood disorders. Patients should consult their doctor if they have a fever or sore throat or any sign of infection while taking this drug.

SSRIs

The initials SSRI stand for serotonin specific re-uptake inhibitors. These work in the same way as tricyclics (see p.60) – they stop neurotransmitters being taken back up into the cell that released them. However, they only work on one type of neurotransmitter – serotonin.

They are effective antidepressants and have fewer side-effects than tricyclics. They are less sedative, do not cause weight gain and do not affect the heart as much as tricyclics. As with tricyclics, caution is necessary in people with epilepsy, and they can cause stomach problems initially. Diarrhoea, nausea and vomiting can occur, as can headache, restlessness and anxiety. These drugs are much safer than tricyclics if taken as an overdose.

SSRIs have not been around for as long as tricyclics. Many specialists believe that they are no better than tricyclics and, as they are very expensive, will only prescribe them for people who cannot take a tricyclic.

There has been much media hype about one drug – Prozac (fluoxetine). This is an SSRI that works very much like the others but has been popularised in some best-selling books. It has been called the 'happy pill' because it has got the reputation of making people with mild depression happier. As it has few side-effects it has been pre-scribed to people with mild depression who

Serotonin Specific Re-uptake Inhibitors (SSRIs)

● Fluoxetine

● Fluvoxamine

● Paroxetine

● Sertraline

● Citalopram

probably may have got better with lifestyle changes alone. Currently in the USA there are many doctors worried about what they see as the over-prescription of this drug. Other SSRIs have similar functions and are just as effective as Prozac.

Some Side-effects of SSRIs

- Stomach problems
- Diarrhoea
- Nausea
- Vomiting
- Headache
- Restlessness
- Anxiety

MAOIs

These drugs (monoamine oxidase inhibitors) were the first antidepressants to be developed. They increase the amount of neurotransmitters in the synapse by stopping them being broken down by a substance called monoamine oxidase. They irreversibly stop the action of monoamine oxidase. Unfortunately, they also work in the rest of the body where monoamine oxidase has some important functions.

One of these functions is to break down a chemical called tyramine, which is in a number of foods. Too much tyramine causes high blood pressure and a violent throbbing headache and can lead to a stroke. As a result, anyone who is taking these drugs must stick to a strict tyramine-low diet and carry a card with them.

It takes two weeks for the body to make new monoamine oxidase and so it takes two weeks for your body to get back to normal after you have stopped taking monoamine oxidase inhibitors. As a result of this you have to stay on the diet for this time; if the drugs have not worked, you may not be able to try another anti-depressant drug during this two-week period.

There is a newer type of MAOI called a RIMA – reversible inhibitor of monoamine oxidase subtype A. There are two types of monoamine oxidase – type A

Monoamine Oxidase Inhibitors (MAOIs)

- Phenelzine
- Isocarboxazid
- Tranylcypromine
- Moclobemide (RIMA)

and type B. As RIMAs inhibit only one type, there is less of a problem with tyramine-containing food, so the diet is less strict. RIMAs block the action of monoamine oxidase but they do not destroy it. The body does not have to make new monoamine oxidase, so the effects are 'reversible' and wear off a day after stopping the drug.

MAOIs are used if a tricyclic or an SSRI has not worked, but some doctors use them from the start in people with depression with reverse physical symptoms, and they may also be used in people whose depression does not fit into any of the well-recognised patterns.

OTHER ANTIDEPRESSANTS

L-Tryptophan This is thought to work by increasing the amount of neurotransmitter made by the brain cells. It is a chemical found in the diet that is turned into serotonin. It is a weak antidepressant but can be used in conjunction with other antidepressants.

Flupenthixol This drug is used for other psychiatric illnesses but is a good antidepressant when given in low doses. It is relatively safe when taken as an overdose and has few side-effects. However, if it is used for a long time, there can be serious side-effects and it should therefore only be used short term.

Nefazodone This works as an SSRI but has fewer side-effects on the stomach. It is better at helping sleep than most SSRIs.

Venlafaxine This is an antidepressant that works like an SSRI. It can cause a skin rash and this should be reported to a doctor immediately because it may indicate a serious allergic reaction. Like many anti-depressants, it may affect the performance of skilled tasks, such as driving.

Reboxetine This drug selectively inhibits the uptake of one neurotransmitter, noradrenaline.

Liothyronine This is a hormone used in the treatment of people whose thyroid gland is underactive. In specialist centres, it may be used in conjunction with other treatments for people with severe depression.

MOOD STABILISERS

These drugs are rarely used to treat depression; they are used to prevent it from coming back by keeping your moods stable if you are prone to depression.

LITHIUM

Lithium makes our cells and our moods more stable. People who have manic–depressive illness are less prone to breakdowns if they take lithium. It also prevents depression in people who suffer severe recurrent depression. It can stop relapses altogether or make them shorter and less severe with longer intervals between them.

Lithium has to be taken regularly and has to be at the right level in the blood. Too little does not work and too much causes side-effects and can be life-threatening. The amount of lithium that needs to be taken by any individual can only be worked out by blood tests.

Before starting lithium, blood tests will be taken to make sure that your kidneys are working properly and the chemicals in your blood are correctly balanced. You will be examined and a heart trace will be taken to make sure that your heart is working properly. The

Stopping Antidepressants

Antidepressants should not be stopped without taking professional advice because withdrawal symptoms may occur.

WORDS OF ADVICE

- Do not stop antidepressants suddenly – they must gradually be tailed off; consult your doctor first.
- Some people who have taken antidepressants regularly for weeks suffer withdrawal symptoms.
- Withdrawal symptoms can be avoided by gradually reducing the dose of antidepressant over a period of about four weeks.

WITHDRAWAL SYMPTOMS

- Nausea, vomiting, going off your food.
- Headache, light-headedness, chills.
- Poor sleep, panic, anxiety, restlessness, mania.

CHANGING ANTIDEPRESSANTS

- Any change to your antidepressant drug treatment should only be done by a doctor.
- Some antidepressants should not be taken at the same time – they are potentially lethal when taken in combination. You therefore have to let one anti-depressant leave your system completely before you start taking another one.
- The changing process may take between one and five weeks, depending on which antidepressant you are stopping and which you are starting.

action of your thyroid gland will also be tested. If there is evidence of disease of the kidneys or of the heart you may not be able to take lithium.

Once you start lithium, blood tests will be taken at least every week until the dose is settled and then every month for three months. After this doctors differ: some take blood tests every two months, others less regularly.

Anything that could make you seriously dehydrated, such as going on holiday to somewhere very hot, diarrhoea, vomiting or starting a new drug (such as water tablets) may alter the amount of lithium you need to take. In this case, a blood test will have to be done urgently.

If you are to have an operation you should tell the doctor you are on lithium because the drug treatment may have to be stopped.

Side-effects of lithium therapy may include tiredness, passing more water than usual, a fine tremor of the hands, a dry mouth and a metallic taste in the mouth. Many of these pass with time. These side-effects should not be confused with signs that the level in your body is too high. If you have severe shaking of the hands, weakness, diarrhoea, vomiting and confusion, see your doctor or go to an accident and emergency department urgently. You may be suffering from lithium toxicity.

Long-term side-effects include weight gain, and lithium can also sometimes affect the thyroid gland. As a result of this, some of the blood taken to test the level of lithium will be sent off for thyroid hormone checks twice a year. Low thyroid hormones can be treated by stopping the lithium or by giving thyroid hormone tablets.

Lithium can affect the way your kidneys function once it has been taken for a while. It can cause you to pass a lot of water and may give you a terrible thirst. If this happens, you should see your doctor and you may have to stop taking the lithium.

Lithium in pregnancy Lithium can harm the growing baby in the early stages of pregnancy, so anyone who is on lithium and plans to have a child should see their doctor and arrange to stop taking the drug. You can start again after three months because the placenta offers some protection to the baby and the baby is then less sensitive to lithium, but this must be done under the supervision of a doctor. The lithium level must be monitored closely because the amount that is needed changes as the pregnancy goes on. More blood tests will be needed than usual. After birth the baby is not protected by the placenta; lithium gets into the breast milk and can affect the baby, so women on lithium cannot breast-feed.

CARBAMAZEPINE

This is another mood stabiliser. It can be used with lithium or instead of lithium in people who cannot take lithium for one reason or another. Blood tests are taken at least every two weeks for the first two months, and less frequently thereafter. Fever may be an indication of blood problems caused by carbamazepine, and so you should consult your doctor if you experience such difficulties.

SODIUM VALPROATE

This is a drug that is used for epilepsy and has mood-stabilising functions. In the past, it was used only if neither lithium nor carbamazepine could be given, but now it is the preferred drug of some specialists. Blood tests should be taken regularly.

OTHER MOOD STABILISERS

Specialists may use drugs that are used in brain conditions such as epilepsy and which have been shown to have a mood-stabilising action, such as nimodipine, lamotrigine, gabapentin and topiramide. The hormone thyroxine is also sometimes used in people with rapidly changing high and low moods. These drugs are used only if more common treatments, such as lithium, carbamazepine and sodium valproate, are ineffective.

ELECTROCONVULSIVE THERAPY

Electroconvulsive therapy (ECT) is one of the most controversial of psychiatric treatments. It is also one of the most effective. It works, and works quickly, in the vast majority of people (eight out of 10) when it is properly prescribed. It has also been proven to be safe.

ECT is usually offered to people whose depression has not responded to antidepressants, people who have medical conditions that mean they cannot take anti-depressants or people who are so severely depressed that they are endangering their life (say by not eating or drinking at all). Some doctors offer it to women who are suffering very severe postnatal depression because it starts working straight away and means they can get back to bonding with their child.

Some people who have had ECT before and on whom it works well have it as an outpatient, but most people stay in hospital as an inpatient.

The idea of convulsive therapy fills some people with disgust. Critics cannot understand why psychiatrists use such a severe treatment. They say that no one knows how ECT works, that it causes permanent problems in the brain and that it is like a form of mediaeval torture and

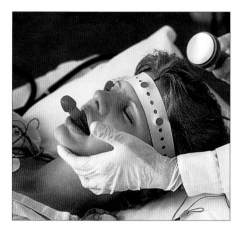

RECEIVING ECT
Although many people have a negative opinion of ECT, it has proved to be highly effective and safe.

has no place in 20th century medicine. The simple truth is that if it did not work, and work well, it would not be used. Psychiatrists are doctors whose duty is to their patients. It is true that no one knows how ECT works, but there are many treatments that doctors give for all sorts of illnesses that they do not fully understand. Studies have shown that it does not cause long-term brain problems. Although some people have complained of some temporary memory loss, modifications in the way ECT is given have reduced this. Most people have no memory loss at all and nearly everyone finds that their memory improves as their depression lifts.

ECT does not solve the underlying problems that caused the depression, but it does return you to a state in which you can start looking at these problems. Like taking drugs for depression, ECT will not guarantee that you will stay well. If you have serious depression you are at risk of a further bout.

WHAT HAPPENS IN ECT?

An anaesthetist gives you a short-acting anaesthetic to help you sleep and something to relax your muscles. Oxygen is given by facemask while you are asleep. A small electric current is passed through your brain using electrodes placed on the scalp. The amount of current given is one-tenth that which is used to start someone's heart if it has stopped. If there was no anaesthetic or muscle relaxant you would have a short fit but, because of the anaesthetic, all that is seen is some twitching of the toes that lasts a few seconds. This is an indication that the brain has a fit but the body does not. You will wake up 10–15 minutes later. Some people complain that their memory is not so good or they feel slightly confused straight after ECT.

ECT starts to work straight away; most people feel significantly better after a couple of weeks. Most people have six to 10 treatments over the course of a few weeks (two to three treatments a week).

GETTING ECT

Written consent is needed for ECT, just as it is for an operation. If you do not consent it will not usually be given. It can only be given against your will if your life is in danger. Your GP, a specially trained social worker and a psychiatrist must all agree that it is required. Then, an independent psychiatrist from the Mental Health Commission will be called in to assess the case. This psychiatrist also has to agree that ECT is required before it can be given, and heor she specifies how many sessions can be given. However, if waiting for this psychiatrist to arrive could be dangerous for you, the doctors can start treatment.

KEY POINTS

- Your GP should be the first port of call when you need help.
- Some brief talking therapies have been shown to work well in depression.
- Long-term psychotherapy tries to sort out long-standing depression; it may not lift your depression in the short term.
- Antidepressants are an effective treatment.
- Antidepressants are not addictive.
- Side-effects of antidepressants can be lessened by starting with low doses or using newer antidepressants.
- ECT is given only to people who desperately need it.
- ECT is a safe treatment for depression.
- ECT does not lead to brain damage.

Women and depression

Women are twice as likely as men to be diagnosed with depression. There are a number of possible reasons for this. For example, it may be just a reflection of the fact that women are more likely to admit to their feelings than men.

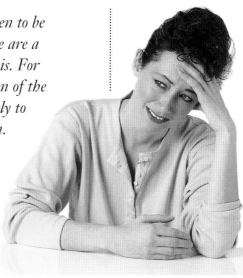

PRONE TO DEPRESSION
Hormones may be one factor in explaining why women suffer from depression more commonly than men.

Alternatively, it may be that male doctors see women as being more prone to depression and so diagnose it more often, or it may be just a reflection of the fact that women go to the doctor more often than men, so doctors have more chance to diagnose depression.

All of these are important factors, but there are also physical differences between men and women that seem to make women more prone to depression. The most important of these is the levels of the sex hormones oestrogen and progesterone. Women have a higher level of these hormones and the levels change during the menstrual cycle, throughout pregnancy and childbirth and at the menopause. The pill, which contains sex hormones, can be a cause of depression.

MENSTRUAL CYCLE

Levels of progesterone and oestrogen vary through the menstrual cycle. Progesterone is only produced for 10 days before a period and then its level drops. It has been implicated as a cause of premenstrual syndrome (PMS, also known as premenstrual tension), which usually begins a few days before the start of menstruation and usually ends shortly after the onset of menstruation – some symptoms of PMS stop as soon as the period begins. Not all women have the same symptoms of PMS but tender breasts, abdominal distension, irritability, anxiety and depression are particularly common.

Some doctors believe that PMS symptoms are the result of changes in progesterone levels, others believe they are caused by worry. They claim that women who badly want a baby may be hoping that their period will not come, and women who do not want a baby hope that their period comes. Both will be worried during the time leading up to their periods. However, these psychological theories have never been proved!

Treatments used for PMS include hormone therapy and water tablets (diuretics), but they often do not work very well. Support and understanding work best in most cases, and treatment is given only to people with severe symptoms. Some specialist NHS centres treat people with severe PMS – occasionally with dramatic improvements.

PMS and the Menstrual Cycle

Premenstrual syndrome, with symptoms that include depression, may be linked to levels of progesterone production.

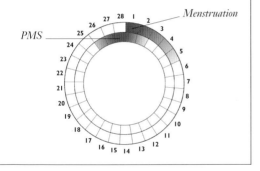

DEPRESSION AND MOTHERHOOD

The levels of oestrogen and progesterone are very high in pregnancy and drop dramatically after the birth. This sudden change can sometimes trigger depression. About half of all new mothers go through the maternity or baby blues, 15 per cent get mild to moderate postnatal depression and one in 500 experiences severe depression.

MATERNITY BLUES

Half of all new mothers suffer from 'maternity blues' in the week after the birth. It is usually around about the third day after the birth that a new mother may start to feel a bit irritable and weepy. Usually she will be back to her old self again by the end of the first week and all she needs in the meantime is support, love and understanding.

AN EMOTIONAL TIME
In the first week after the birth of a baby, many mothers suffer 'maternity blues', but these pass in a few days.

MODERATE POSTNATAL DEPRESSION

Long-term depression is common after childbirth. It often goes unnoticed as it is put down to the new mother adjusting to her responsibilities or being kept awake at night. The severest types of depression occur soon after the birth of the baby, but the least severe and most common start between two weeks and a year later. Sometimes depression starts around the time when the support and attention of friends and family begins to wane. The symptoms may be more vague than in other types of depression. Often the woman is very anxious, especially about whether her baby is well and feeding properly, and she may seem to be full of guilt and self-criticism as well as constantly tired and irritable.

The Risk Factors of Postnatal Depression

Certain factors increase the likelihood of the new mother suffering from postnatal depression. The more risk factors that a woman has, the greater her chance of depression.

BEFORE THE BABY IS BORN

- Fertility problems
- Past psychiatric illness
- Psychiatric illness in the family
- Single parent
- Serious financial problems
- Having a child when very young (under 16 years)
- Having a child when over the age of 35
- Uncertainty whether you want the baby or not
- Worries about the baby's health
- Mild to moderate anxiety during the last three months of pregnancy
- A difficult labour

AFTER THE BABY IS BORN

- Preterm birth
- Physical illness
- Social isolation
- Lack of support from your partner
- Returning to work at a lower level of seniority

Postnatal depression cannot be explained simply by hormone changes. For one thing, the major changes in hormone levels often occur long before the depression begins. It may be that they make a woman prone to depression, but social factors are important too.

In general, you are at increased risk of postnatal depression after a particularly difficult pregnancy or birth, when the reality of motherhood or the change in role fall below expectations and/or when having a new baby brings relationship difficulties to the fore.

Treatment is usually needed for postnatal depression. A recent study showed that both antidepressant drugs and cognitive–behaviour therapy (see p.54) are effective. Most antidepressants can be taken while breast-feeding.

When a woman is being treated for postnatal depression, it usually helps if her partner can become involved and understand what is happening. In some cases, fathers may be in need of support too: there is a high risk of depression in new fathers who have depressed partners.

Treatment makes a big difference to recovery rate: women who get treatment for postnatal depression are likely to get completely better, while those who do not have a 50:50 chance of feeling better by the child's first birthday.

SEVERE POSTNATAL DEPRESSION

A more unusual type of postnatal depression affects a minority of women who become severely depressed in the first two weeks after birth. It is more likely after the first pregnancy, in those who have had a psychiatric illness before and in those who have psychiatric illness in the family. It is thought that hormonal changes may act as a trigger for depression in those who are prone to it.

In severe depression, a woman loses touch with reality and she may have delusions and hallucinations. There is a real risk to her baby in this situation, and mothers who are severely ill have been known to kill their babies. Some depressed women believe that the world is so bad that they should put their child out of its misery, whilst others believe that there is something wrong with their child and that they are performing a mercy killing. When the situation is as serious as this, the woman will probably have to be admitted to hospital for treatment, especially if there is a risk that she might harm her baby or herself. The ideal place is a hospital mother and baby unit, where she can be with her baby and have help from the staff to care for him or her.

Treatment is usually with antidepressants, and the mother may also have other types of medication to deal with hallucinations and delusions.

It is usually possible to breast-feed while taking medication, but small amounts of drugs do get into the breast milk. When a high dose of medication is required, or if the baby is particularly sensitive to the drugs, it may be necessary to switch to bottle-feeding if no other medication is suitable. A mother who is being treated with lithium (see p.65) will have to stop breast-feeding as babies are very sensitive to its effects.

Some doctors offer electroconvulsive therapy for severe depression after childbirth. It works quickly and enables the new mother to get on with bonding with her child. The vast majority of women are treated with tablets.

If you have postnatal depression you are likely to make a good recovery, but you will be at risk of developing depression after any future pregnancies. You should tell your doctor or obstetrician that you have had postnatal depression before you have your next baby so that you can be monitored and receive early and prompt treatment if you need it.

THE MENOPAUSE

Women are more likely to seek help for depression around their middle years. Many doctors believe that this is due to the menopause. The theory is that hormone level changes spark depression as they can do after childbirth or with premenstrual syndrome. However, there is no reliable evidence that depression is actually more common at the time of the menopause.

There are, of course, a number of other changes that often happen in many women's lives in middle age and that may play a role in triggering depression. For example, their children may leave home, their relationship with their partner may change or their own parents may become ill.

In the UK, women who have a depressive illness and happen to be around the time of the menopause will be treated with antidepressants if appropriate, just like anyone else with a similar condition.

However, in the USA psychiatrists are more convinced that hormones are the cause and some prescribe treatment with oestrogens. It is unclear whether this works, but some women in this country who are prescribed hormone replacement therapy (which includes oestrogen) for menopausal symptoms say that they feel less depressed while taking it.

AFTER OPERATIONS

Research from some years ago claimed that women were more likely to become depressed after either being sterilised or having a hysterectomy, but recent research has cast doubt on this.

The ovaries produce a number of hormones whose functions are not clear, and some doctors in the USA say that, in some women, their removal will cause depression. Other doctors say that hysterectomy sets off depression only in a woman who is already predisposed to psychiatric illness, while some experts point out that there are some women who actually recover from psychiatric symptoms after a hysterectomy.

The same applies to sterilisation operations. In other words, it may be only those women who were at risk of depression in the first place who will develop the illness after being sterilised.

WOMEN AT HOME

Women may have a higher rate of depression because of their social situation rather than because of anything to do with their hormones. In a landmark study, researchers in south London surveyed women who were at home during the day. They found that those most likely to be depressed were young mothers with three or more children under ten, with an unsupportive partner, with no one else to confide in, who were poorly housed and who had no employment outside the home.

UNDER PRESSURE
The demands of several small children, combined with difficult social conditions, can trigger depression.

KEY POINTS

- There are many reasons why women are diagnosed with depression more often than men.
- Changes in oestrogen and progesterone levels may trigger depression.
- Depression after childbirth is often missed but can be treated effectively.

Grief and bereavement

There is a complex link between bereavement and depression. Bereavement can trigger a depressive illness, although it usually does not. A recently bereaved person can experience many symptoms that are similar to depression.

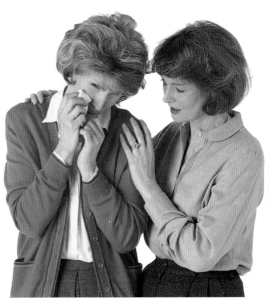

In one study, about 30 per cent of recently bereaved widows over the age of 62 were found to have symptoms of depressive illness. In bereavement, suicidal thoughts, mental and physical slowness and worry about past actions are much less likely to occur. If you suffer from these you may be depressed rather than just grieving. If you have thoughts of self-harm or you completely stop eating you should see a doctor urgently.

SUPPORT IN GRIEF
Everyone needs someone to talk to when they are grieving, but if grief triggers depression then counselling may be necessary.

NORMAL GRIEF

Grief is a normal experience; it is painful but it does not require medical treatment. There are three stages of normal grief that can be distinguished.

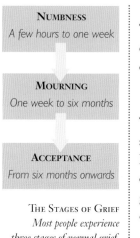

NUMBNESS
A few hours to one week

MOURNING
One week to six months

ACCEPTANCE
From six months onwards

THE STAGES OF GRIEF
Most people experience three stages of normal grief, although the intensity and length of each stage varies from person to person.

NUMBNESS

This lasts from a few hours to one week. You may feel emotionally numb and feel as if the person has not died or that you cannot accept the reality of their death.

MOURNING

This lasts from one week to six months (easier after about three months). You may feel sad or depressed, have little appetite, find yourself crying a lot, be agitated or anxious and have little concentration. Some people feel guilty. They feel they had not done enough for the deceased.

Others blame professionals or friends and family. You may find that you have physical symptoms such as pain during this phase. Most people have the feeling at some time during this stage that the deceased is present in some way, and one in ten report seeing, hearing or smelling the person who has died when they are obviously not there. Many of the experiences mimic depression but they are normal – you are not depressed or going mad.

ACCEPTANCE

This takes place from six months onwards. Symptoms subside and you accept the death and try to get back to normal. This takes a variable length of time.

COPING WITH GRIEF

Grief is natural and so are your feelings. Grief is a process that has to be worked through. If it is not, then feelings could fester and they could catch up with you in the end, turning into depression. Grief should not be bottled up and needs to be let out. Even if you seem to be having a severe reaction to the death at first, you are likely to come through the process with just the support of your friends and family or a counsellor.

It is usually best to turn to your family and friends initially. They may often need to grieve themselves, and the help and support that they offer you will help them to come to terms with what has happened. You are not a burden, it is a two-way thing. They need you as well.

Counsellors can offer support in grief and can help people work through the process in a controlled way. They are particularly useful if you find that you are not passing through the stages of grief or you are having a particularly difficult time. Bereavement counsellors aim to help you acknowledge the death by helping you to talk about the circumstances surrounding it; they encourage emotional expression of the pain of grief; they try to identify coping strategies and people who might offer support; they help the process of building a new life and help you let go of the dead person. You can contact such counsellors through your GP, or ring CRUSE or other self-help groups listed in 'Useful addresses' (see p.91).

THE BEREAVED

Giving space for a grieving person to talk about their feelings is all important. Most people think that they need to say how wonderful the deceased was, but that is often not the support that people need. They need space to talk about how they feel. They need to be allowed to say how bad they feel, how distressed they are, how they might feel guilty or angry that they have been left behind, how they said something bad before the person died and how the death brings their own mortality closer. All these thoughts and feelings are normal and need expression.

Causes of Intense Grief

Although the death of a loved one is always hard to bear, certain situations make the grief even more intense.

- If the death is sudden or unexpected
- If the death results in blame for the survivor
- When a parent's child dies
- When a young child's parent dies
- When an adult was dependent on the person who died
- When the survivor has difficulties expressing their feelings
- When the survivor is currently still adapting to a previous loss
- When the survivor is socially isolated
- When the survivor has dependent children

MEDICATION FOR GRIEF

Medication can be counterproductive early on in the grieving process. Though drugs may make you feel better they may interfere with the process of grieving and prolong it. It is painful to work through the feelings of loss, but it is the only way to get back to normal.

If you really cannot sleep at all for the first few days your GP may prescribe tranquillisers. This will only be for a few days to help you sleep, and then they will be stopped. In extreme circumstances these may be useful for a few critical days but should not be used long-term. Though they may help you to feel better, they will not help you work through your grief and you will have to do this when you stop taking the tablets. It is only if grief turns into depression that drug treatment has any place in the long term.

ABNORMAL GRIEF

Not everybody passes smoothly through the stages of grief. Some people find that they do not pass through the normal stages and suffer persistent problems. Others find it difficult to grieve and do not acknowledge the death at all. Some people find that they are consumed with intense anger or feelings of betrayal which last for months. If grief is intense and unbearable it needs to be treated. Contact your GP or counsellors such as those at CRUSE.

KEY POINTS

- Grief is a normal reaction.
- Medication is not usually needed and may be counterproductive.
- Self-help organisations can provide excellent bereavement counselling.

Helping friends and family

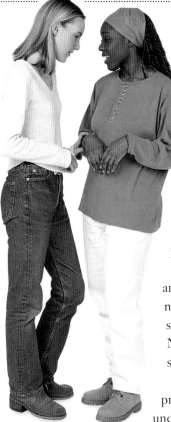

If you are able to recognise when someone is depressed and offer support, your help will be priceless. You may not think that you have done very much, but you will have helped someone in need and may even have helped prevent a suicide.

A Friend in Need
It is not always easy helping a depressed friend, but the support that you can offer may prevent a suicide.

Many people who are depressed find it difficult to take up offers of help, so do not be put off. Try to be patient and tell them that you are ready to talk when they want to.

When you do talk, be sympathetic, be supportive and try to convince them to see their GP. There is no point telling a person who is depressed to snap out of it or to pull him- or herself together. Nobody likes being depressed, and he or she would snap out of it if possible.

Talking allows people to work through their problems, but listening is not easy. It can be uncomfortable, especially when someone you know is distressed and saying things that are either not true or so painful that you do not know how to cope with the emotions they produce in you. Know your limits and do not take on too much.

Try not to give quick, ungrounded reassurance or quick advice and do not think you have to say something because you feel uncomfortable. Do not jump in and interrupt – give them time and space to say what they feel. Accept that they feel the way they do and see the world the way they do. If you think they are wrong, explain why you think so and give them proof, but do not get into an argument. You will be doing a good job if you listen, acknowledge how the person feels, are sympathetic and hold back on giving too much advice.

Remember, you can assure them that medical treatment is effective and that they will get better.

Once you have talked things through, try to keep in touch, be accessible and offer practical help and support until they are better. Helping people to get help by offering to accompany them to a GP appointment can be useful, but be careful not to take over. Many people with depression feel ineffective, and taking over their decisions may make them feel worse.

PREVENTING SUICIDE

Of the 5,000 suicides in England and Wales each year about 3,000 are the result of depression. The box on p.90 lists groups of people who are at high risk but it should be borne in mind that anyone who is seriously depressed may be thinking about suicide, and you should be vigilant. Attempts at suicide are not just a way of getting attention and they should always be taken seriously. Of course there are people who try to harm themselves as a cry for help – but if that cry goes unheard, goes wrong or is in the context of depression then it could herald suicide.

If You Feel Suicidal

If you feel suicidal, **seek help**. Speak to someone urgently. Talk it over with your partner, a friend, your GP, the Samaritans – anybody.

Knowing about depression, ensuring that someone who is depressed gets treatment and keeping in touch are all important. Supporting someone who is suicidal without professional help is very difficult. If you are at all worried you should try to convince the sufferer to see someone as soon as possible. They can go to their GP or into any accident and emergency department, or it may be possible to arrange for a doctor or nurse to come to see them at home. Your local psychiatric department may have an emergency clinic that you can just walk into.

HELPING A SUICIDAL FRIEND

If you suspect that a person is suicidal, talk with them and let them speak about their feelings. Ask them if they have ever thought it was not worth going on. Some may say yes and that they have thought of taking their own life; others may say that they have not thought of it but they have gone to bed at night hoping that they would not wake up. Both groups of people are potential suicide risks.

Of course some people intent on suicide will deny that they have thought of it; you may have to judge whether they are telling the truth. Many people find speaking about their suicidal impulses is a tremendous release and it may actually stop them going through with suicide.

If you do not live with them, make sure that they have your telephone number and the number of their GP, the Samaritans and other caring agencies. Arrange a definite time when you will see them again. This could be in an hour or two or the next day depending on how they are. If you can get their agreement to remove paracetamol, large quantities of antidepressant or non-essential drugs from their medicine cupboard, this would be a good move. If you are worried that your friend is in imminent danger, do not leave them while you are getting in contact with caring agencies if at all possible.

It is always best to discuss what you are doing with the sufferer. They will probably agree that they should see someone, but if they do not and you really think that they are a danger to themselves, you should act in their interests. If you think you should, contact the GP, the Samaritans or their family. You can contact the local psychiatric outpatients and see if there is a walk-in clinic, or take them to an accident and emergency department.

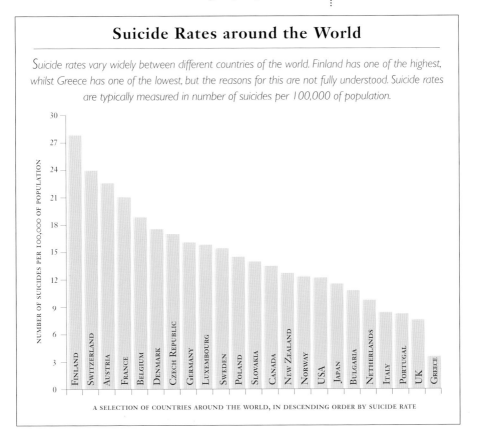

Suicide Rates around the World

Suicide rates vary widely between different countries of the world. Finland has one of the highest, whilst Greece has one of the lowest, but the reasons for this are not fully understood. Suicide rates are typically measured in number of suicides per 100,000 of population.

A SELECTION OF COUNTRIES AROUND THE WORLD, IN DESCENDING ORDER BY SUICIDE RATE

Factors that Increase Suicide Risk

The likelihood of a person committing suicide is increased if any of the following conditions or categories apply to them.

- Severe depression
- Serious physical illness accompanying depression
- Person has spoken about suicide
- There has been a past suicide attempt
- There has been a suicide in the family
- Continuing severe life stresses such as divorce or bereavement
- Person is lonely and socially isolated
- Person is male (and therefore more likely to succeed in his suicide attempt)
- Person is unemployed
- Person takes illicit drugs
- Person has alcohol problems

KEY POINTS

- Listening may be the most important thing that you can do for family and friends who are depressed.
- Anyone who thinks about suicide should contact their GP, the accident and emergency department at their local hospital or the Samaritans, and get help.
- Depression can be treated – you will feel better.

Useful addresses

Association for Postnatal Illness
25 Jerdan Place
London SW6 1BE
Tel: (020) 7386 0868

British Association of Counselling
1 Regent Place
Rugby
Warwickshire CV21 2PJ
Tel: (01788) 578328

Compassionate Friends
53 North Street
Bristol BS3 1EN
Tel: (0117) 9645202
Helpline: (0117) 9539639

CRUSE Bereavement Care
Cruse House
126 Sheen Road
Richmond
Surrey TW9 1UR
Tel: (020) 8940 4818
Helpline: (020) 8332 7227

Depression Alliance
35 Westminster Bridge Road
London SE1 7JB
Tel: (020) 7633 9929

Depressives Anonymous
36 Chestnut Avenue
Beverley
East Yorkshire HU17 9QU
Tel: (01482) 860619
Fax: (01482) 876334

Lesbian and Gay Bereavement Project
Unitarian Rooms
Hoop Lane
London NW11 0RL
Tel: (020) 8455 8894/8200 0511

Manic Depression Fellowship
8-10 High Street
Kingston Upon Thames
Surrey KT1 1EY
Tel: (020) 8974 6550
Fax: (020) 8974 6600

MIND (National Association for Mental Health)
Granta House
15–19 Broadway
London E15 4BQ
Tel: (020) 8519 2122

National Childbirth Trust
Alexandra House
Oldham Terrace
London W3 6NH
Tel: (020) 8992 8637

National Phobics Society (NPS)
407 Wilbraham Road
Manchester M61 0UT
Tel/Fax: (0161) 881 1937

Relate
National Office
Herbert Gray College
Little Church Street
Rugby
Warwickshire CV21 3AP
Tel: (01788) 573241

Royal College of Psychiatrists
17 Belgrave Square
London SW1X 8PG
Tel: (020) 7235 2351

SAD Association
PO Box 989,
Steyning BN44 3HG
Tel: (020) 8969 7028

The Samaritans
46 Marshall Street
London W1V 1LR
Tel: (020) 7734 2800

Nearly 200 branches across the country. 24-hour service every day of the year. Local branches listed in telephone book.

Saneline
Tel: 0345 678000 (14:00-24:00)
Offers support and information and has details of local services.

Terence Higgins Trust
52–54 Grays Inn Road
London WC1X 8JU
Tel: (020) 7831 0330

Triumph Over Phobia (TOP UK)
PO Box 1831
Bath BA2 4YW
Tel: (01225) 330353
Fax: (01225) 469212

Index

Acknowledgements

PUBLISHER'S ACKNOWLEDGEMENTS
Dorling Kindersley would like to thank the following for their help
and participation in this project:

Editorial Assistance Alyson McGaw; **Design Assistance** Paul Jackson, Chris Walker;
Production Michelle Thomas; **DTP** Jason Little;
Consultancy Dr. Sue Davidson; **Indexing** Indexing Specialists, Hove;
Administration Christopher Gordon.

Illustrations (p.58) ©Philip Wilson

Picture Research Andy Sansom; **Picture Librarian** Charlotte Oster.

PICTURE CREDITS
The publisher would like to thank the following for their kind
permission to reproduce their photographs. Every effort has been made
to trace the copyright holders. Dorling Kindersley apologises for any
unintentional omissions and would be pleased, in any such cases,
to add an acknowledgement in future editions.

Hulton Getty p.16; **Image Bank** p.7 (Romilly Lockyer), p.26 (A. Boccaccio); **Rex Features** p.8;
Science Photo Library p.22 (Biophoto Associates), p.29 (NIBSC), p.3 & p.31 (BSIP, Krassovsky),
p.41 (Oscar Burriel), p.48 (Claire Paxton and Jacqui Farrow), p.55 (National Library of Medicine);
Tony Stone Images p.17 (Donna Day), p.34 (Chris Craymer).

AUTHOR'S ACKNOWLEDGEMENTS
The author would like to thank Dr. Deirdre O'Gallagher for her helpful
comments on the text and Dr. Natasha Crowcroft, Alexander McKenzie
and Nathaniel McKenzie for their patience and support.